Behind the Mask:

*The Mystique of Surgery and the
Surgeons Who Perform Them*

by David Gelber, MD

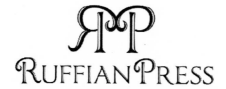

RUFFIANPRESS

Ruffian Press
150 FM 1959
Houston, TX 77034
www.ruffianpress.com
www.itpfuturehope.com

Library of Congress Catalog Number: 2011901707

ISBN-13: 978-0-9820763-5-4
ISBN-10: 0-9820763-5-5

First Edition – 2011

Cover Design:
Duncan Long
www.duncanlong.com

Typesetting/Book Layout Design:
Gianna Carini
www.brighteyes.org

Printed in the United States of America.

Dedication

This book is dedicated to the memory of Anthony Dibene-detto, Chief of Surgery at Nassau County Medical Center for many years. "The Chief" taught me to think like a surgeon and, by word and deed, demonstrated the dedication that every surgeon must have to his patients and to his craft.

Behind the Mask:

The Mystique of Surgery and the Surgeons Who Perform Them

by David Gelber, MD

Table of Contents

IV. The Lighter Side

I. Preoperative

The Surgeon's Prayer

"Dear Lord, please protect me from the interesting cases and don't let me screw up today."

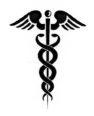

1. Introduction

*B*ehind the Mask: The Mystique of Surgery and the Surgeons Who Perform Them takes the reader on a journey through the mind of a surgeon; presenting a viewpoint
that touches on the triumphs and failures surgeons face every
day. The book presents a series of essays that progress from
preoperative considerations to the intraoperative experience
and finally to the postoperative perspective. I have tried to
make it accessible to the non-medical reader as well as the
physician or nurse. There is a glossary of terms that I hope
will be helpful and I have tried to explain the medical terms
and conditions as plainly as possible.

Surgery, presented from the surgeon's perspective, is
something most people, including many non surgical physicians, never get to see or read about. The unexpected twists
and turns that a patient can take after even the simplest
procedure presents a challenge that mandates constant vigilance by the surgeon and his staff. At the same time, sometimes a surgeon knows, by having just rooted around inside
a patient, that everything will be okay. Training, experience,
insight, knowledge, and more than a touch of humility com-
bine to create a surgeon.

Each chapter examines a particular aspect of surgery; they are loosely arranged with an introductory section, a section dealing with preoperative considerations, followed by the intra-operative experience and, finally, postoperative considerations. The final section takes a look at the lighter side of surgery and medicine. All the anecdotes and patient scenarios presented are true to my best recollection, but all the names have been changed. I hope these pages will help remove some of the mystery that surrounds the practice of surgery. I hope the reader comes away with new understanding of what it means to be a surgeon and, perhaps, to be a patient.

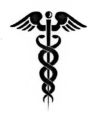

2. On Surgery

Surgeons must be very careful
When they take the knife!
Underneath their fine incisions
Stirs the Culprit—Life!
　　　　　—Emily Elizabeth Dickinson

For more than twenty years I have made my living as a general surgeon, spending hours, almost every day, rummaging around inside people's bodies. This is more than a job, perhaps even more than a profession; it is best described as a passion. The surgeon is called to be passionate about what some would call the unthinkable, the extraordinary, the epitome of arrogance. "Arrogance," one may ask. "How can that be?"

What a surgeon does can only be called arrogant. He or she takes an incredibly sharp instrument, proceeds to slice through living human tissue, and in the course of the operation decides what organ is offensive and is to be removed, and what is innocuous or important and is allowed to remain. Or, the surgeon may rearrange our tissues, taking what was once God's perfect creation and altering it for a presumably nobler purpose.

Man nobler than God? Impossible. Such is the arrogance of the surgeon.

Of course, I don't in any way imagine any man, surgeon, priest, baker, or used car salesman to be nobler than God. It is one of the consequences of living in this fallen world that we need surgeons. Diseases and the specter of Death, having been released with the first taste of the forbidden fruit, create a need for physicians and surgeons to help keep these evils at bay.

What is it that makes anyone do such a thing? How is it that out of a typical class of one hundred medical students some will choose a career in surgery? And, after years of rigorous training, of getting out of bed at three in the morning to attend to an anonymous individual who had the misfortune to be hit by a bus, shot, stabbed, suffer a perforated intestine, or any number of maladies that can't tell time; this endeavor remains a passion, something done for the reward of seeing the sick and injured walk out of the hospital alive and whole.

I've frequently thought that what surgeons do for a living would be reason for incarceration if it was done away from the operating theater. In general, cutting people open with sharp objects is considered socially inappropriate and frowned upon by legal authorities. To avoid this hazard the operating theater was developed and we surgeons try to limit such endeavors to that location. Theater is an appropriate description; surgery used to be performed in just such a way. Students and professors would observe the operation from seats in an amphitheater; sterility not a prime concern in those days. Even after the research of Joseph Lister introduced the concept of asepsis to surgery, thus eliminating the open spectacle, the operating room still had observation decks, frequently seen in old movies, but rare today.

So, we surgeons, haughty actors of the medical world, ply our trade before a smaller, but captive audience: anesthesiologist, circulating nurse, surgical technician, surgical assistant, and the occasional student. But, the star and center of any operation is not the surgeon; rather it is the patient. Above all, the patient is given the greatest attention, loving care with every detail of the procedure geared towards carrying this individual to a successful outcome.

Before any operation, time is spent evaluating, examining, and explaining the operation to the patient. A very common question I hear is something like this: "This is routine, isn't it?" Most of the time the answer is that a particular operation is common, hopefully straightforward, but I never consider it routine. Every operation requires proper planning, attention to detail, and the utmost care. And, with every procedure, surgeons have a single goal; to perform the right operation, at the right time, with proper technique so that our patient returns to their normal life as expeditiously as possible.

A general surgeon spends 5-6 years in residency, after medical school, studying and practicing every aspect of the profession so that at the end of his time he believes he is fully and properly trained. This residency provides the necessary basics; how to evaluate a patient, plan surgery, carry out the operation and provide post-operative care. All those years certainly seems to be enough time to learn all that needs to be learned. But, in reality, the practice of surgery is a lifetime of learning. Every day brings the potential for something new, an unexpected anomaly, a new presentation of an old disease, a situation never previously encountered; one that may only echo a vague memory of an article read in an old journal.

So, in our arrogance, we are humbled. It is this humility that separates the good and very good surgeons from the great surgeons. Because, every person that picks up a scalpel has to have the arrogance, the confidence that says I can do this better than anyone. If this belief is missing and the surgeon believes that another surgeon can do the job better, then it is in that patient's best interest to be referred to that other surgeon. If humility is lacking, the patient may suffer.

What about humility? Physicians quickly learn that, despite our best therapeutic efforts, the human body can be a frustrating and unforgiving subject. Invasion by micro-organisms, tumors, external forces, and foreign objects or even the body attacking itself can rapidly overcome all our good intentions. We do all we can to give our patients the greatest chance for complete recovery and, happily, we are successful in the vast majority of cases. But, every individual is unique and every individual demands our unflagging attention. It is something I am reminded of everyday. The truly great surgeon is never so arrogant as to believe that something can't be wrong. It is an unfortunate truth that patients sometimes become sick after surgery; that our best efforts may not have been good enough. When this happens we start to look for a reason; all this searching usually leads back to the original operation; something bleeding or not healing as expected, an infection, or a wide variety of other potential complications. And so, it is the surgeon's humility that allows him or her to say, "Something's not right, I need to figure this out and solve this dilemma." It is this attribute that comes with experience and is the single, most difficult thing for the young surgeon to learn.

Arrogance and humility, truly an oxymoron, but no two words give a better description of what we surgeons are made of. It takes a truly unusual, dedicated person to follow the trail that at the end bestows the title, "Surgeon." I have followed this path for twenty years and have always enjoyed the challenge. I hope you are informed and entertained by the words presented on these pages.

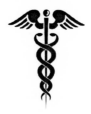

3. Changing Times

Medical science has made such tremendous progress that there is hardly a healthy human left.
—Aldous Huxley

From trepanning, which is drilling holes in a patient's head to release evil spirits, to therapeutic bleeding to amputations, the practice of surgery has existed, in one form or another, for thousands of years. It was frequently a brutal practice, one where the cure was sometimes worse than the disease, where the quality of the surgeon was measured in seconds and the only sure outcome was a wound spewing forth "laudable pus" that might eventually lead to a survivor.

But with the discovery of microorganisms, asepsis, and anesthesia, surgery moved from the dark ages into a modern light. The work of Joseph Lister, who pioneered the concept of sterility; William Morton, an American dentist who first reported the use of anesthesia; Louis Pasteur, who discovered microorganisms; William Halsted, who instituted many innovative surgical concepts including rubber gloves, and many others led to the modern practice we now call surgery.

I've been thinking about how medical knowledge and practice has changed over the twenty-five years that I've been a doctor. I recall a lecture I heard during my second year in medical school, given by one of the pathologists. She stated that autopsy findings on deceased patients revealed that the clinical diagnosis was incorrect almost sixty percent of the time. What this meant was that sixty percent of the time the patient was being treated for the wrong condition.

I thought this statement was astounding and more than a bit disturbing. Think about it: The supposedly most brilliant minds of the day were wrong more than half the time. That fact made us little better than ancient and medieval physicians whose "cures" often were worse than the disease. I wasn't sure that I believed that pathologist, and I would be very surprised if she could give that same lecture today.

The amazing advances in imaging and interventional techniques over the last thirty years have greatly improved diagnostic accuracy. CT scanners, MRI's, PET scans, endoscopy, laparoscopy, and other new and emerging technology, utilized in various combinations, provide incredible visualization of previously obscure "black boxes."

The abdomen has always been one such hidden entity. When I was in medical school, 1980-1984, CT scanners were just coming online. If we had a patient that was ill and the Chief Resident decided that an abdominal CT scan was necessary, he would tell the intern to order a CT scan of the abdomen; the intern would then delegate to the medical students on service the task of getting the test scheduled. No problem, one might think; put the order in the computer and the test gets done. This is true for 2010, but in 1982 it was necessary to fill out a requisition, hand carry it to the radiology resident, grovel for fifteen to twenty minutes begging that the scan be approved, and then find out it would be done on Thursday, three days hence.

The scan would routinely take about 1½ hours to finish, all the time the medical student forced to stay and "babysit" the sick patient, whether it was at 7:00 a.m. or twelve midnight. I soon learned to befriend the unit secretary, who seemed to have miraculous powers and invariably was able to schedule the test the same or the next day and at a convenient time, well worth the price of a box of doughnuts.

Times slowly changed. During residency, CT scans were done much more expeditiously, usually the same day. During my Chief Resident year, a new CT radiologist was hired who believed, like I did, that using CT scans to evaluate the abdomen was good medicine. The information obtained unlocked the hidden world of the abdominal cavity and diagnostic accuracy soared. From trauma, to diverticulitis, to appendicitis, CT scans provide a wealth of information that would have been unavailable in 1980.

For example, one of the measures of the quality of a general surgeon used to be his or her accuracy in diagnosing acute appendicitis. Until fairly recently, this disease was almost exclusively diagnosed on clinical grounds, that is, history and physical exam. Indeed, the most useful medical book I ever read was one called *Cope's Early Diagnosis of the Acute Abdomen**. This very concise book offered a practical approach to the patient presenting with abdominal pain. In a very clear and informative manner it carried the reader through the steps necessary to determine what the potential etiologies of various abdominal maladies could be. Appendicitis, cholecystitis, intestinal obstruction, and a host of other intra-abdominal conditions are covered. The information I learned from that book remains one of the most useful tools in my arsenal.

However, the days of depending solely on the history and physical exam to diagnose appendicitis, or any medical condition, seem to be gone. Now, if I am called by an Emergency

*William Silen, MD, *Oxford University Press*, 2010

Room physician about a patient with abdominal pain, and acute appendicitis is suspected, I will usually be told a cursory history; physical findings will often be omitted and there will be an accompanying CT scan report almost 100% of the time. Often the report will merely state "acute appendicitis" and sometimes the report will be wrong.

So, we have progressed from diagnosing appendicitis on clinical grounds with about 85% accuracy to diagnosing it utilizing radiologic criteria with about 85% accuracy. Of course, combining the two diagnostic modalities increases the accuracy tremendously so that I would say the diagnosis of acute appendicitis is now about 98% accurate when all the available investigative tools are employed.

Another remarkable change in surgery over the years is the shift from inpatient procedures with long post-operative convalescences to outpatient procedures with short hospital stays, rapid recovery, and return to normal activity in days or weeks instead of months.

Once again, appendicitis is a prime example. In medical school, patients with acute appendicitis would usually undergo emergency surgery as soon as the diagnosis was made. However, diagnosis often required a period of observation in the hospital that varied from a few hours to a few days. The operation was done with a standard open "McBurney" incision utilizing muscle splitting technique, and then the patient spent 5-14 days in the hospital and would be limited in their activity for about six weeks.

Contrast this past scenario with today where the patient presenting with abdominal pain is rapidly diagnosed and taken to surgery within a few hours of presentation; is often discharged the following day; and is back to normal activity in about five days or less.

Even greater changes are apparent for cholecystectomy, which is removal of the gallbladder. In 1980 such an operation usually entailed admission to the hospital the day before surgery with exposure to potential antibiotic resistant pathogens that have colonized most hospital wards; a six-inch incision below the ribs or in the mid-abdomen, an NG tube (tube going through the nose into the stomach), a drain at the surgical site exiting through the abdominal wall, and 7-10 days in the hospital.

Over the years, all of these have passed into oblivion, eliminated from routine elective cholecystectomy. The NG tube was probably the first to go. Indeed, such tubes have been found to be unnecessary for most elective abdominal surgeries. Admission on the day prior to surgery disappeared in the 1990s as almost all patients scheduled for elective procedures are now admitted the same day. In fact, insurance companies and Medicare require a very compelling reason for a patient to be admitted the day before surgery.

The routine use of drains faded away in the 90s and the advent of laparoscopic surgery made the operation completely ambulatory.

Now, a patient undergoing cholecystectomy can expect to be admitted to the ambulatory surgery unit one to two hours before surgery, have their thirty-minute operation, spend a couple of hours in the recovery room, be discharged home to sleep in their own bed, be back on a regular diet within twenty-four hours, and back to work in five to seven days, if not sooner.

Another amazing advance is the capability of operating successfully on older and sicker patients. I remember, as a third-year medical student, seeing a patient with multi-organ system disease. He was in his seventies, diabetic, with coronary artery disease, hypertension, a cigarette smoker, but otherwise in "perfect" condition. He was diagnosed with severe, life threatening colitis causing severe systemic sepsis (overwhelming infection) and needed immediate emergency surgery to have any chance of survival. My reaction at the time was, "What's the point? The patient has so many medical problems, he'll never survive a big operation."

Of course I was wrong, even for those times. However, in this day and age, there would never be any question about operating on such a patient. A patient in his seventies with such comorbidities is not unusual these days when we routinely perform surgery on octogenarians and even nonagenarians. Seventy is almost considered to be a spring chicken and even with the associated chronic illness this patient could expect to live five, ten, or even twenty years more.

The change is as much a product of attitude as resources and technology. Thirty years ago such a patient with significant chronic illness suffering from a surgical condition such as chronic gallbladder disease or hernia would have limited choices. Mostly, he or she would have to learn to live with the discomfort or inconvenience. Even though surgery had emerged from the dark ages of the 1800s, it was still frequently considered to be an option of last resort, to be used when all the proper medical, non-operative modalities had failed. I remember Internists stating that it was their lot in life to "save" their patients from the surgeon. Such an attitude is rare today. Well coordinated care of patients with clear, open lines of communication between the team of physicians attending to these patients that have multi-organ disease is the norm, at least in the community hospitals where I practice. I can't speak for academic centers; in the past there always seemed to be a bit of animosity between Medicine and Surgery.

Patient expectation is the main driving force behind a lot of the changes I have noticed. In this day and age any patient capable of thinking independently wants to live a full life, free of pain and disability. Recurrent pain caused by gallbladder disease or the discomfort and limitations that may be associated with a groin hernia are unacceptable, particularly when there are safe, ambulatory procedures that can relieve even a minor degree of suffering. In such cases, the potential morbidity is weighed against the risks and the decision is reached jointly with the patient and family, who are, hopefully, fully apprised of all the potential risks and benefits.

Minimally invasive procedures with ultra modern intraoperative monitoring make even the sickest patients candidates for surgery if the procedure has appropriate, proper indications. Of course, that last phrase, "appropriate, proper indications," is most important and this necessity is one thing that hasn't changed. During my residency we had a weekly "indications" conference; every resident went through every procedure that they had performed and presented the indications for the surgery to the attending staff. The importance of having the proper indications for any procedures, and that such indications were adequately documented, was drilled into the brains of the resident staff. Even today, as part of every procedure that I consider, I review the indication in my head. If I am not sure that the reason to perform a certain procedure is clear, then I will reconsider and look for alternatives.

Over the years it has become clear that surgery done with shaky or inappropriate indications invariably leads to complications or poor outcomes. Removing a gallbladder that is not diseased often leaves the patient with diarrhea that may or may not resolve. The patient with a sick gallbladder, however, usually has minimal or no side effects from cholecystectomy. This is because a truly sick gallbladder usually does not function normally and, in a patient with chronic symptoms, the biliary tract and digestive system have had time to compensate and adjust so that removal of the diseased organ causes little change in the patient's digestive physiology, except that their symptoms disappear.

By far, the greatest change in the last thirty years is the development and widespread implementation of minimally invasive procedures, be they laparoscopic, arthroscopic, endoscopic, or endovascular. More being done with less is the truly great leap in surgical care. We haven't quite reached "Star Trek" levels where Dr. McCoy merely had to wave his medical tricorder over Chekhov's head to make the diagnosis of epidural hematoma and then wave another device to repair the damage, but the advances since I've become a surgeon have been remarkable.

Laparoscopy was the province of the Gynecologist when I was in medical school; no respectable General Surgeon would stoop to such levels. But, in the late 1980s, coinciding with the development of higher definition video cameras and monitors, techniques for laparoscopic general surgical procedures were developed. Operations that used to require hospital stays of several days or longer could now be done on an ambulatory basis. Cholecystectomy, appendectomy, repair of hiatal hernias, and many other abdominal and pelvic operations became less painful, with less disability, and rapid return to normal activity.

Along with this change came a change in attitude. The idea of "protecting" the patient from the surgeon seems to have disappeared. Patients who would never have been considered for surgery in the past are now referred without trepidation. Indeed, patients with extensive comorbidities, who have been told that they couldn't withstand a major surgery are able to tolerate these minimally invasive procedures.

So, indications have changed. In vascular surgery, caring for patients with blockages in arteries, usually going to the leg, endovascular procedures allow relief of symptoms that patients previously had to learn to live with. Such operations have always been among the most complicated and high risk. Balloons and stents have replaced scalpels and sutures so that even the sickest patient can be freed from pain and disability, and limbs that used to end up in the trash can now be revascularized and healed.

So, we've come a long way from the old days of a fast and dirty operation, followed by routine infectious complications and severe morbidity. Who knows what the future will bring?

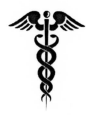

4. *The Rules*

1. Never cut anything if you don't know what it is.

2. If a blood vessel has a name, it deserves to be tied twice.

3. Never open the Common Bile Duct unless you are sure it is the Common Bile Duct.

4. If a patient wishes to have a second opinion, wants a different surgeon, a different hospital, or wants to cancel their elective surgery, always comply.

5. If you think a patient is not going to heal well, they probably won't; perform the operation accordingly.

6. If someone offers help, accept it.

7. Treat the pancreas with all the respect it deserves and stay away from it whenever possible.

8. Taking shortcuts in surgery always ends up costing much more time in the long run.

9. Operations done without proper indications always come back to haunt you.

10. If complications develop after surgery always look to the surgical site for the causative agent.

11. Always follow numbers 1-10.

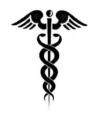

5. *Fearfully and Wonderfully*

I praise you because I am fearfully and wonderfully made; your works are wonderful, I know that full well.
—Psalm 139:14

Psalm 139 declares that we are fearfully and wonderfully made. Over the course of more than twenty five years spent caring for a wide variety of sick and injured bodies, I have come to agree with the profound truth of this statement. The human body is constructed in a remarkable way that keeps it running during the most trying situations.

From the top of our heads to the soles of our feet our bodies are constructed to withstand extremes of temperature, assaults by invading organisms, physical and mental challenges, and to perform with uncanny accuracy under the most arduous and taxing conditions.

So, let us start with the bottom of our feet. The plantar aspect or soles of our feet are a thick layer of skin and fascia perfectly suited for the stress and strain of upright walking. All the trumpeting of modern technological advances in athletic shoe design has not yielded any product that can claim to be superior to our feet. Indeed, recent research suggests that running barefoot or with a flat shoe with minimal padding is far superior to the thick-soled, complicated athletic shoes that probably create more stressors for our feet than they prevent. It seems that Hobbits had it right.

Our bodies are maintained at a near constant temperature, 98.6 F or 37.5 C. We are equipped with very efficient heaters and coolers to keep us in the appropriate narrow range. If our body temperature starts to rise, be it secondary to a hot environment, physical exertion, or some other factor, we will sweat (or perspire, if you are a lady). The moisture can cool directly, but the greatest cooling is a result of evaporation from our skin. External adjuncts, such as fans, speed the process. Rapid breathing can also contribute to elimination of heat via the lungs. Of course this is carried to an extreme in dogs, who pant to cool themselves.

Conversely, our body is constantly producing heat. Routine, but essential metabolic processes all generate heat. In a cold environment this metabolism speeds up and more heat is generated, often manifested by shivering. Similarly, in the course of many illnesses, a patient develops a fever. In the most extreme circumstances an ill patient will develop uncontrollable shaking called "rigors." Such shaking is the result of rapid muscle contractions designed to generate heat and rapidly raise body temperature. In such situations the "thermostat" is turned up. Body temperature rises from the normal 98.6 to 101 or 103 or even higher. During the rising phase the patient complains that he feels cold and will attempt to cover himself to conserve body heat until the new temperature set point is reached. Although such high fever is a cause for concern and does carry its own set of risks, there seems to be some benefit, aiding our body's fight against invading pathogens.

The fever may persist or it may dissipate, at which time the patient will usually have profuse sweating, that lowers body temperature, as the fever "breaks." The fever must play a role in repelling an invasion by micro-organisms. The higher body temperature seems to have an inhibitory effect on certain viruses and bacteria. In the post operative patient, fever is very common. Low grade fever, below 101.5, is probably secondary to a systemic inflammatory response unrelated to infection. Above this level, there is more concern that an infection might be present.

In any scenario, the fever has a purpose, be it fighting infection or assisting with the healing process and is one example of the amazing intricacies of human physiology.

Fever, of course, is a very common occurrence, be it a simple cold or life threatening sepsis. There is an aspect of human physiology and anatomy that is very important to our well being. Our bodies are built with long tunnels passing into and through us. The aerodigestive tract allows us to exchange a variety of elements with the outside world. The tracheobronchial tree starts at a shared entrance with the digestive tract. In the pharynx, the two systems divide, with the respiratory limb ending in the lungs, two balloon-like structures that constantly inflate and deflate, exchanging inhaled oxygen for carbon dioxide, a byproduct of cellular metabolism. This essential mechanism keeps us alive. In fact, the first two letters of the ABC's of trauma resuscitation are Airway and Breathing, (the third is Circulation), the jobs performed by the lungs.

But, it is the efficiency of our lungs and airway in light of constant bombardment by potential pathogens from the world around us that is truly remarkable. Our upper airway is equipped with mucus membranes that secrete mucopolysaccaride chemicals that trap invaders so they can be expelled or killed. Our upper airways are also outfitted with cilia, tiny hair-like structures that rhythmically beat and carry foreign particles away from the lower bronchial tree. We have the ability to cough, an extremely efficient mechanism that clears uninvited strangers from our lungs and trachea. Finally, our alveoli, the tiny balloons where gas exchange occurs, have all the components of our immune system standing at readiness to attack any invaders that make it to that level. Should this final line of defense be overwhelmed by bacteria, viruses or merely large particles, infection and/or impairment of gas exchange occurs. Pneumonia results from micro-organism infection of the lungs. Smoking damages cilia and allows particulate matter to reach the ends of our airways, eventually causing damage that is irreversible, the common condition called Chronic Obstructive Pulmonary Disease (COPD).

The other fork of the aerodigestive tract leads to the esophagus, stomach, and the small and large bowel. While the lungs are efficiently scavenging wayward invaders, the gastrointestinal tract has learned to live in harmony with such organisms. Technically, the GI tract lumen is outside our bodies. It is a long, tortuous tunnel that snakes its way from our mouth to our anus. Inside this tunnel trillions of bacteria reside in a symbiotic relationship; welcome, as long as they stay in their place.

The numerous types of bacteria play a crucial role in maintaining normal physiology and immune function. It is likely that the resident bacteria stimulate a variety of immune functions, particularly during the early developmental years. The bacteria help with digestion of certain nutrients, breaking down complex polysaccharides into more digestible forms and also play a key role in the enterohepatic circulation of bile salts. In addition, the GI flora help with the absorption of certain vitamins and play a protective role for their human host by preventing the overgrowth of harmful bacteria within the gut lumen. As long as these tiny helpers stay inside the tunnel of the GI tract they are our friend. If they escape and invade surrounding organs or spaces, then they are most unwelcome. But, the normal GI tract physiology is a wonderful example of symbiosis between vary disparate organisms.

It is easy to see that the human body is an amazing creation that is well suited to living and flourishing in a hostile world. But what is it that sets the human apart from other animals. Other animals may run fever and are also bombarded by microscopic invaders. Is there anything that sets the human apart; an attribute that screams: "I am unique to the Homo sapien; you won't find me in a dog or a chimpanzee"?

GK Chesterton said it was art that separates humanity from all the rest of creation. The ability to paint, write, sculpt, play, or write music is the sole province of mankind. The ability to appreciate such endeavors is an even greater exclusive human attribute.

But what is it that allows a Bach to write music that soars, a Picasso to create unique, expressive paintings or a Charles Dickens to string together a series of words that actually make sense and have the power to entertain and inform? There are two components of the human body necessary for such creation. The first and most obvious is a brain, an organ that is incredibly complex, with mechanisms that are poorly understood, but capable of the most astounding achievement. Every original thought, every idea that became a concept and then a commodity started in the recesses of someone's brain.

A mass of neurons, synapses, electrical impulses, and chemical transmitters work in harmony to produce a thought. This thought may be the next logical conclusion from a series of previous thoughts or it can materialize from nowhere, an inspiration from an unseen Muse. Thoughts may be fleeting or they may coalesce into ideas. Eventually the idea comes to fruition and a new creation emerges. Humanity lurches forward into new realms with every thought and idea. Unfortunately, some ideas seem to cause us to step back.

The passage of idea to commodity requires that some form of work be performed and the principle agent of such work, particularly in the arts, but also in most other endeavors is the hand.

A complex organ made up of skin, bones, nerves, blood vessels, and muscle, the hand is capable of turning black and white notes on a page into the sweet sound of Rachmininoff's Piano Concerto Number Three; it can mold and shape a lump of stone into Michelangelo's David. This incredibly versatile organ allows us to surpass all the rest of creation, to create the art that we all appreciate.

It is possible to provide substitutes for our hands; amazing creations have come from people who have lost the use of their hands. But, as we marvel at the human capacity to adapt to such disability, consider what these talented individuals could have done. Substitutes for our hands can be fashioned or trained, but they remain substitutes, at best performing nearly as well as a normally functioning hand, but never surpassing the hand.

A whole book could be written on the amazing design of the human body. Many of the intricacies are still being discovered, but it is this remarkable design, this body so perfectly suited to thrive in the world that surrounds us, that allows someone like me to slice a patient open from stem to stern, root around inside for a while, stitch the wound closed, and then see that patient walk into my office a month later entirely well. Truly amazing.

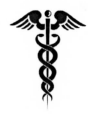

6. The Watchdog

Watchdog

1. A dog trained to guard people or property.
2. One who serves as a guardian or protector against waste, loss, or illegal practices.

Have you ever wondered why, in years past, people didn't always die if they developed appendicitis or intestinal perforations or any of the intra-abdominal maladies that continue to plague us today. I do a large number of surgeries for these and other similar problems; I find it hard to believe that before abdominal surgery became fairly routine everyone died if they developed such surgical emergencies.

Watchdog is defined as "a dog kept to guard a property" or "a watchful guardian." Our bodies have all been built with such a watchdog. God, in his infinite wisdom, created us with a marvelous, but unsung organ called the omentum. Never heard of it, you may say. Most people outside of medical circles are oblivious to the existence of the omentum, but to those of us who make a living grouping around people's insides, this amazing organ keeps us and our patients out of trouble.

What's the omentum? Almost everyone has this organ, but it is almost never mentioned in high school or college textbooks on anatomy. We all learn about the liver and pancreas and our intestines, but the omentum is the guardian to all these vital organs. Just inside our abdominal cavity, lying like a curtain draped over our intestines is the omentum. Structurally, it is a sheet of fat, blood vessels, and lymphatic tissue that literally is an apron providing a protective cover to our abdominal viscera.

Most of the time all it is called to do is lie dormant, ever vigilant, but quiescent. However, when the need arises, it springs into action. There have been numerous times I've operated on a patient and followed this remarkable organ to the exact location of the offending process. It seems to have a sixth sense that causes it to move in and seal off diseased areas in our abdominal cavity. Invading bacteria are kept isolated, and what could have been a massive infection, becomes a localized and relatively minor annoyance.

Take, for example, diverticulitis, which is a very common condition these days. Diverticuli are small protrusions that can develop on our colons where the inner lining of the colon bulges through the outer muscular coat, akin to the inner tube of a bicycle popping out of the outer tire. These diverticuli can become inflamed and rupture, which allows the bacteria inside the colon to leak out into the abdominal cavity. A catastrophe and life threatening emergency, one would think. However, here comes the omentum to the rescue. Like the "Blob" of movie legend, this organ will adhere to the area of perforation, sealing the hole and preventing potential life threatening spread of the contaminants. The diverticulitis often is diminished to a minor episode of pain in the lower abdomen, frequently treated successfully with oral antibiotics as an outpatient.

I've had patients come to see me with symptoms typical of appendicitis that have been present for nearly a week. Normally, appendicitis that has been ongoing for such a time would have developed an abscess or severe peritonitis. Yet, there is the patient, sitting up, smiling with only minimal discomfort. What do you think is found at surgery? A very nasty, inflamed, gangrenous appendix with the omentum encircling it like a gift wrapped present waiting to be delivered to the proper recipient, in this case, me, the surgeon.

The omentum has been described as an organ that brings new blood supply to areas in need. In fact, it is often utilized for just such a purpose. Plastic surgeons may use it to reconstruct areas damaged by cancer, radiation therapy or severe infections. When I encounter a difficult intestinal problem, a difficult perforation or something similar, I frequently use the omentum to help remedy the situation. And, when it is absent, having been removed or utilized for some other purpose, I am hardpressed to find a suitable substitute to replace this remarkable organ.

It must be true that in the days before modern surgery, the "watchdog" saved many lives. Inflammatory processes leading to abscesses and often death have been described since the time of Hippocrates. Often these patients died of their disease, but many recovered uneventfully. It is almost certain that these recoveries were due to our marvelous omentum. It is no wonder that general surgeons call the omentum their best friend and ally. It has truly earned its title, "The Watchdog."

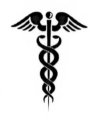

7. Talking to Patients

The doctor may also learn more about the illness from the way the patient tells the story than from the story itself.

—James B. Herrick

Years ago I read an article about what patients could or should expect from a visit to their doctor. There were four patients that recounted their experiences during recent doctor's appointments. The length of time they had to wait, the details of their visit including actual time spent with the doctor were included. One of the patients complained that the doctor spent most of his time talking to her. I would bet that this particular doctor was the most thorough and conscientious of all the doctors that were presented in that article.

When a patient walks into a doctor's office for the first time, the doctor faces a myriad of possibilities. In my general surgery practice, I usually assume a new patient has or is suspected of having a surgical problem. Of course this differs from the primary care physician setting where the problem could be anything from headache to hemorrhoids. It is the primary care doctor's task to sort out all the endless possibilities and determine the best medical approach for each. This is their great challenge, one that may be faced twenty times a day or more.

Fortunately for me, the surgeon has a task that is a bit easier, at least initially. When I am asked to see a new patient, most of the time there is some information that comes with the request, usually something short and simple, ie: Gallbladder disease, abdominal pain, cold leg, etc. This very brief summary gives me a bit of direction, although occasionally it can lead in the wrong direction.

So, the first, and often the most useful, thing that I do is to sit and talk to the patient. Probably 98% of the time the patient will tell me what's wrong and all that I need to do is confirm this presumptive diagnosis with the physical exam and appropriate testing. This is true for almost any condition, be it acute appendicitis or hemorrhoids.

But, how does simple talking do all this? The things that go through a doctor's head, at least mine, when I take a history from a patient, are myriad. First and foremost is, "Is this patient 'sick.' " By this I mean does the patient seem to have a severe, possibly life threatening condition that warrants immediate hospitalization and possibly emergency surgery? Patients that cannot sit up, are afraid to move, or are unable to give any history because they are too ill usually need to be in the hospital. It is one of my unwritten rules that patients that look sick usually are. Experience teaches doctors, particularly general surgeons, to be vigilant, assume the worst and do all that we can to achieve the best outcome.

But, I've strayed from the point of this article. Talking to patients is the single most important part of patient visits. When I went to medical school the greatest amount of time was spent on learning the natural history of the many various diseases, all the possible presenting symptoms and signs and how to obtain this information from a sick patient. Unlike *House*, I don't believe that patients always lie. Most want to get better and most of the time the questions that I ask cannot be answered in a misleading way. Starting with the simple question, "What brought you in here today?" and then paying attention to the patient's answer, will, in a few minutes, provide almost all the information necessary to begin that individual on the road to recovery.

Approaching a patient with abdominal pain provides an excellent example. In the days before routine CAT Scans the evaluation of patients presenting with abdominal pain required the skills of a detective; the history and physical exam, along with limited diagnostic testing, were the mainstays of diagnosis. The abdomen, in the days before high resolution CAT scans and MRI's, was a black box filled with vital organs and often inaccessible except through surgery.

The abdomen is usually divided into three segments, epigastrium, which is above the umbilicus (belly-button), mid-abdomen, the level of the umbilicus, or hypogastrium, which is below the umbilicus. The first thing I will usually ask is, "Where did your pain start?" Sometimes I get an answer like, "In the bathroom"; some people are so literal. But, once properly directed, the starting point of the pain will go a long way to narrowing the choices for the offending organ.

Epigastrium usually means stomach, duodenum, gallbladder, liver, or pancreas. Mid-abdomen refers to the small bowel or the right side of the colon and hypogastrium usually refers to the left colon. These divisions are in no way arbitrary, rather they correspond to the nerves that supply the various organs and where the nerves will refer pain. For instance, the gallbladder sits in the right upper abdomen, but very often gallbladder pain is felt in the middle. This is because the visceral nerves refer the pain to the middle. Only after a gallbladder becomes more inflamed do the more specific parietal nerves come into play and the pain then becomes localized over the offending organ.

Duration, quality and associated symptoms all direct me to a working diagnosis that only needs to be confirmed. Physical exam, blood/urine tests, and imaging studies are used to confirm the working diagnosis and to eliminate other possibilities. I've learned that relying solely on imaging studies is often misleading.

For instance, just recently I was called from the Emergency Room at one of the hospitals and informed of a patient that the admitting physician wanted me to see in consultation. The ER physician said she had right-sided abdominal pain and that an ultrasound had revealed gallstones. The white blood cell count was elevated, but she was otherwise stable. This patient, as presented to me, was properly admitted to the hospital, but a patient with these clinical findings generally is not a life and death emergency and can usually be seen later in the day. It is very rare for uncomplicated cholecystitis (gallbladder inflammation) to require immediate surgery.

I saw the patient a few hours later and the history that I received led me to very different diagnosis. Her pain was in the right lower abdomen, unusual for gallbladder disease, and she said it was very severe. She also had a history of severe cardiac disease. There was associated nausea and constipation. Physical examination revealed severe tenderness in the right lower abdomen and no tenderness in the right upper abdomen, where the gallbladder usually resides. I began to be concerned that she could have had appendicitis, which would require emergency surgery. The other possibility I considered was ischemic colitis (inflammation of the colon caused by poor blood supply), also a serious condition that could be a life threatening emergency.

When I checked the tests that had been done I saw that a CAT scan had also been done, which seems to be almost routine these days. The findings were thickening of the cecum, which is the first part of the colon, and a normal appearance of the appendix. With all this information, I determined that the patient likely had ischemic colitis, but that surgery was not necessary at that time. The following day she had a colonoscopy which definitively confirmed the diagnosis and she is now recovering; responding to the non-operative therapeutic regimen that was started. She still has her gallbladder and her asymptomatic gallstones.

What is apparent is that properly talking with the patient, obtaining a clear history, points the physician in the right direction. Talking to patients is a skill that is easy to develop and actually saves time and money. It often takes no more than five minutes to gather the most pertinent history from a sick patient and, as I've shown, the rest of the workup flows out from this relatively short, but very informative interview.

So the next time you go to your doctor and he or she spends most of your appointment talking to you, be thankful; thankful that you have a doctor that cares enough to take the time to find the right answer in the right way.

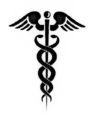

8. The Villain

Man is a creature composed of countless millions of cells: a microbe is composed of only one, yet throughout the ages the two have been in ceaseless conflict.

—A.B. Christie

Performing surgery and taking care of surgical patients presents many challenges, rewards, and pitfalls. The greatest of these challenges and the biggest pitfall is the battle against infection. From the time of the first hole that was drilled into a skull up to the latest stereotactic operation, infection has been the evil villain lurking in the shadows.

The first surgeries relied upon the speed of the surgeon, the manifestations of infection were common and expected; the germ theory, Pasteur, and antisepsis were unknown. Infection after surgery was routine and the surgeon, following the established teachings of Galen, waited for the thick "laudable pus" that indicated a localized infection, rather than the universally fatal signs of systemic sepsis.

In the 1890's, William Halsted, practicing at the newly established Johns Hopkins Hospital instituted surgical protocols that required strict asepsis, meticulous surgical technique, sterilization of instruments, and the first use of rubber gloves. Of course, his use of rubber gloves was strictly for the protection of his favorite surgical nurse, whose hands were irritated by the caustic mercuric chloride that was used to cleanse the hands prior to an operation. Halsted continued to operate barehanded for sometime, refusing to accept the diminished tactile sense associated with wearing gloves.

Today, strict asepsis, gowns, masks, caps, and gloves are mandatory for all but the simplest surgical procedures. Instruments and equipment are all sterilized and any break, or even suspected break, in proper technique requires taking appropriate corrective action. Every effort is made to fend off the villain and protect the surgical patient. Post surgical infections, ranging from minor, superficial wound infections to disastrous infections of orthopedic prostheses are the great enemy that we surgeons face with every operation.

But, what happens to cause such infections and how can we know that they are occurring? The source of almost every infection is the patient's own, native bacteria. Our bodies are a vast repository of bacteria, most living in harmony with us, but some potentially lethal. Most of the E. Coli living in our GI tract is perfectly harmless, unless it manages to invade the urinary tract or peritoneal cavity. Staph and strep are probably always on our skin, but let them contaminate an artificial heart valve or hip prosthesis and weeks, months, or even years of woe ensue.

So we scrub and paint and gown up; we try to prudently administer appropriate antibiotics and then we stay vigilant. The first sign of infection requires some response. It is at this point that skill and judgment are most needed. The first slight fever that appears post-operatively raises questions; is it merely atelectasis (collapse of a portion of the lung, very common and easily treated) or is it the harbinger of full blown sepsis, a severe, systemic infection. How do we know? Signs and symptoms, caution, and a high index of suspicion are utilized to help dictate the proper response, be it watchful waiting, instituting appropriate therapeutic antibiotics, evaluating with diagnostic studies, or intervening in more drastic ways.

One of the remarkable things about modern surgery is the small number of serious infections that actually do occur. In my practice it is extremely rare to see a post operative infection after elective operations. Ambulatory surgery, proper use of prophylactic antibiotics, maintaining aseptic technique, and appropriate choice of operation all contribute greatly to the low infection rate.

But, what of the surgical disaster, the patient with severe, overwhelming infection, rightly called systemic sepsis. Sepsis; the word conjures up images of a huge septic tank or repository for human waste. And, when a patient develops sepsis, that is what he or she becomes. Bacteria, wherever they may be hiding, send out various chemicals and the body responds. The irony is that it is often this response that causes the most damage. Think about it. If you take a blunt object and drag it over the skin of your forearm, exerting some pressure you will develop a wheal, a swollen, red area that is somewhat tender to touch. Your body has initiated a mild inflammatory response. Fluid pours into the area, blood flow increase and a variety of chemicals are released which "call out the troops," that is, different cells that respond to stress by causing inflammation. If infection by bacteria or other microorganisms is present the response is enhanced.

Now imagine such a process racing through your entire body. Fluid pours out of your circulating blood to bathe all your tissues, the blood vessels dilate to try to increase flow to every cell in your body. The autonomic nervous system assumes a prolonged fight or flight stance, doing its best to maintain perfusion to your brain, heart, and lungs, while shutting down blood flow to kidneys, GI tract, and skin. What does the doctor find in this situation? A severely ill patient with rapid heart rate, low blood pressure, cold clammy skin, rapid respirations, little or no kidney function; in one word: dying.

Such a situation mandates an immediate and aggressive response. Administration of intravenous fluids in adequate, sometimes massive, amounts to restore and maintain circulating blood volume, antibiotic therapy targeting suspected pathogens, supportive measures which may include artificially breathing for the patient via ventilators, instituting dialysis, starting medications that will push a failing heart to do more; in short, starting treatment that will buy time until this deranged body can begin to heal itself and resume its normal function.

While all these supportive measures are initiated a search is made for the underlying culprit. Relatively common conditions are sought, such as infection in the urinary tract or lungs. One of my rules of surgery is that when a patient gets sick after surgery, always look to the surgical site for the cause. Serious wound infection, abscesses, poor healing of intestinal repairs, or anastamoses are often the culprit.

When discovered, such surgical complications present the greatest therapeutic challenge. Complications are always unfortunate and all efforts are made to avoid them, but in this day and age when we operate on ever sicker and more elderly patients, occasional complications are inevitable. However, it is the response and treatment of the complication that is the great challenge. I think that more malpractice lawsuits are won due to inadequate treatment of a complication than for the actual complication. The decision to intervene with another surgery, a simpler drainage procedure by a friendly interventional radiologist, or to maintain aggressive non-operative therapy without additional procedures requires weighing all the risks and benefits and often includes consultation with other physicians.

The critically ill patient almost always requires a team approach. The expertise of various consultants provides the greatest hope for complete recovery. The critical care nurse is another vital cog in the ICU wheel, perhaps the most vital. A study was done several years ago looking at variables that affected outcomes in ICU patients. The only factor that made a difference was the quality of nursing care.

In my own experience I have found this to be true. An experienced critical care nurse that understands the deranged physiology of the ICU patient can make the difference between a complete recovery and death. Subtle changes in patient's condition, such as increased heart rate, fever, changes in sensorium all are warning signs; little bells that ring announcing that the villain is arriving and it may be time to make a change. Vigilance by the medical team is vital when battling such a villain.

There are times when serious, life threatening infections require action in minutes; when the luxury of trying a course of antibiotics or other nonoperative therapy is not an option. Certain, so called necrotizing infections are one such situation, the aptly named "flesh-eating bacteria." Usually, the emergent situation is apparent. The case of James, a patient I cared for about fifteen years ago, sticks in my mind. I was called by James' Internal Medicine doctor to come and see him immediately in the Emergency Room.

James was awake, but very ill. His blood pressure was 60/0, his heart rate was 140. On his left thigh was a patch of black skin about 3 cm in diameter and there was some redness on his right arm. In the course of my three-minute initial evaluation the black area on his thigh doubled in size. I informed him that he needed immediate surgery. His response was that he wanted to think about it and perhaps he would have surgery in the morning. My answer was that if he took that much time to think he wouldn't be around to make a decision.

He was taken immediately to surgery where I started to cut away dead, rotting tissue. The infection had spread between all the muscles of his thigh and I cleaned it up as best as I could. He improved, but remained very ill. Consultation was obtained with a Plastic Surgeon, a specialist that would be most important when James was ready for reconstruction, a stage I hoped he would survive to reach.

Ultimately, he needed two more surgeries to eliminate all the infection and defeat this particularly nasty villain. The Plastic Surgeon and I eventually had to amputate his left leg at the hip; but he survived, recovered completely minus his left leg, and I saw him for other problems several times in later years.

I have seen numerous similar cases over the years; Diane who was similar to James, but pulled through, also losing her left leg; Jeffrey, so tragic, but not because of his infection. His life-threatening infection was fortuitously diagnosed early so that he needed only debridement (removal) of the dead tissue rather than a major amputation.

Jeffrey stands out for a couple of reasons. First, it was only by luck that I saw him fairly early in the course of his illness. I was called to consult on his case, but was told that it was "only cellulitis," a simple infection that rarely requires immediate surgery, and so I made plans to see him on rounds the next morning. A few hours later I was called about another patient that needed immediate attention and so I returned to the hospital and, since I was there, I stopped to see Jeffrey, also.

The other patient was nothing serious, but Jeffrey was a different story. He was young, only in his twenties, and had suffered a minor blister on his foot recently. His most recent lab tests revealed a white blood cell count of over 40,000, extremely high and suggestive of a very serious infection or some other serious underlying condition. It was his foot that really revealed the severe infection. Normally, skin suffering from cellulitis is red and swollen, hallmarks of the increased blood flow to the infected area. Jeffrey's foot and ankle were blue and white, indicative of decreased circulation, very unusual for routine cellulitis.

He was scheduled for immediate surgery; the infection was confined to the skin and all the offending tissue was removed. He avoided any sort of debilitating surgery, needed only a simple skin graft, and returned to his normal life.

About one year later I saw his name on my schedule for an office visit and, at the time, I wondered what the problem was. He missed that appointment and then two more. My office staff called him as is our protocol when patients miss appointments, but they weren't told anything and no excuse for the missed appointments was offered.

About a week after the third missed appointment his father called stating that Jeffrey had died. Needless to say, this was very unexpected. I wondered if it was related to his previous illness, but was informed that he had died of a drug overdose. I was saddened by the news. Whenever someone dies needlessly it is tragic; more so when it is someone young with so many years ahead, made worse by succumbing to our own weaknesses.

I never found out any more details about Jeffrey; I don't know if he had the problem when I first treated him or if it developed after his illness. He and his family never mentioned it and I never saw any signs. Perhaps, I was so blinded by his severe illness, the evil villain that had invaded his foot, that I ignored the larger demon that was tormenting his body. I don't think I'll ever know for sure.

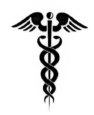

9. Accomplices

The only weapon with which the unconscious patient can immediately retaliate upon the incompetent surgeon is hemorrhage.

—William Stewart Halsted

If infection is the villain, then this particular villain has several accomplices. Surgery is supposed to occur in a strict aseptic environment, the patient should be able to resist infection, have adequate nutrition to heal surgical wounds and have blood that clots in a normal manner. Any deficiency in one of these areas can lead to prolonged post operative recovery, complications, or disaster.

A post operative infection begins with a microorganism contaminating the operative site. Most commonly, such a microbe is a resident of the patient; one that enters the field from the skin or GI tract. Sometimes, the offending beast may come from a break-in technique, a hole in a glove, or improperly sterilized instrument. In a normal patient undergoing an uncomplicated operation, a few bacteria are easily handled by an intact immune system and there is no adverse outcome.

But, in a compromised patient, one with immune deficiency, poor clotting, or poor nutrition, even a tiny amount of contamination can be disastrous. Patients that are elderly, with cancer, liver, or kidney disease, diabetes, AIDS, or a number of other conditions are at risk for major complications and require extra vigilance before, during, and after surgery.

When a surgeon is handed a scalpel and makes a skin incision, the patient's first line of defense is breeched. Bleeding occurs from the skin edges and the wound could fill up with blood if steps are not taken. Most surgeons will pick up the electrocautery and "buzz" the bleeders. In the old days, before the cautery, the surgeon would employ dozens of clamps; clamping and tying each individual vessel with very fine sutures. The late Dr. Robert Sparkman, one of my favorite teachers, used to clamp each vessel, but didn't tie them. After a few minutes he simply removed each clamp and the bleeding was controlled. He relied on the body's ability to clot to stop the bleeding and this maneuver was successful over 99% of the time. Controlling bleeding in this manner, besides being effective, also avoided leaving behind unnecessary foreign bodies. Although sterile, even this tiny amount of foreign material could become a nidus for future inflammation or infection.

Blood clotting is absolutely essential to even the simplest operation. Tiny capillaries and small vessels normally clot after a few minutes in a normal, healthy patient. However, in the patient with a coagulopathy, that is one whose blood won't clot, successful surgery becomes nearly impossible.

For example, there was an operation on Sara several years ago. She was a lady of 84, hospitalized at an LTAC, that is a Long Term Acute Care hospital. Such facilities care for patients that needed prolonged hospital stays for IV antibiotics or more intensive therapies than were offered at the lower level Skilled Nursing Facilities. Sara was having abdominal distention, constipation, and occasional rectal bleeding. Evaluation had revealed a narrowed segment of sigmoid colon, the part of the colon just above the rectum. There was concern that it was a cancer and would continue to bleed. After discussion with her family (she was unable to make the decision), she was scheduled for a colon resection with a colostomy.

Her surgery was very uneventful, lasted about thirty minutes, and she was admitted to the ICU for post operative monitoring. That evening I was called because her blood pressure was low and her abdomen was distended. Her hemoglobin level had dropped. Every indication was that she had significant intraabdominal bleeding and she was returned to surgery. The operative site which had been perfectly dry (meaning: no bleeding) when the surgery was initially finished was now resident to a large hematoma (a collection of blood).

After scooping this blood clot out of the abdomen I looked for the cause, hopefully a solitary vessel that was responsible for ruining my evening. There was a lot of oozing from the areas of dissection, but no single source. When a patient is returned to surgery for post operative bleeding, the surgeon always hopes to find a single vessel that is squirting or oozing blood, tie it off, and be done with it. When a situation like Sara's is encountered, it is a bit disconcerting. In Sara's case, testing of her coagulation status revealed a severe coagulopathy; her blood would not clot. The preoperative evaluation had been normal and there was no indication during the initial surgery that there was a clotting abnormality, but, whatever the reason, her blood would not clot. In this situation there is only one alternative; pack the area with surgical pads to tamponade the oozing and then try to reverse the clotting abnormality. This usually involves finding the cause and correcting it, combined with replacing the necessary factors that are needed to promote a clot. In Sara's case, the cause could not be found, the bleeding persisted, and she eventually died from this complication.

A similar case with a happier outcome was Adam. Adam had been in the hospital for about one week when I was called to consult on his case. He was twenty five years old and had complications secondary to Crohn's disease, an inflammatory condition that affects the bowel. In his case he had multiple intrabdominal abscesses and signs of systemic sepsis: high fever, elevated white blood cell count, and his abdomen was very tender when examined. He was taken to surgery and had removal of the offending segments of small bowel.

He was monitored in the ICU after surgery and, because of his sepsis and also the appearance of his tissues at the time of surgery, I left an order that he was not to be given any anticoagulant therapy. Such treatment, which involves the administration of blood thinners, is common practice in hospitalized patients to prevent blood clots in leg veins. I was concerned that he would have an unacceptable risk of bleeding if any of the commonly used anticoagulants were administered. Despite this order, he was started on Arixtra, a powerful blood thinner.

The next day he was tachycardic (rapid heart rate) and hypotensive (low blood pressure), and his hemoglobin level had dropped. The Arixtra had been ordered by another physician and the nurses had given it despite my order, at the assistance of the ordering doctor. It was obvious that Adam was bleeding to death. Despite the anticoagulation he had received, there was no choice but to return to surgery. He had four liters of blood in his abdomen, more than half his circulating blood volume. It was obvious that his blood was not clotting, so, once I'd cleaned out all the blood, I packed his abdomen.

Happily, Adam had a better outcome. His coagulopathy was corrected and, forty eight hours later, he was returned to surgery, the packing was uneventfully removed, and he was able to leave the hospital about two weeks later.

But, what about bleeding that is less dramatic; small or moderate amounts that are common after most operations? In most cases, this blood is reabsorbed by the body and little or no consequence. Any collection of blood, however, can serve as the breeding ground for unwelcome bacteria.

A collection of blood, called a hematoma, is a barrier to the body's defense mechanisms. White blood cells cannot circulate through the semi-solid mass of coagulated blood. Bacteria, however, if present at the time of the surgery, love to hide and reproduce in such an environment. If I perform an appendectomy and the appendix has ruptured, presumably bacteria are floating around the surgical site. If there is bleeding into that site and a hematoma forms, trapping the unsuspecting, but thoroughly delighted bacteria inside, trouble can start to brew.

The bacteria thrive on the bloody environment, tucked safely away from the vindictive white blood cells. Even with antibiotic therapy an abscess can develop. Of course, this usually takes some time, but it is a common reason a patient will need readmission to the hospital 7-14 days after surgery. And, it is in this way that bleeding from any cause becomes an accomplice to the villain of infection.

The villain's other major accomplice is poor healing. Every surgical procedure requires at least some healing. Surgical wounds breech the body's natural defense mechanisms. After the surgery, despite sutures and staples, the patient must heal the wounds that have been created. Everything that has been mentioned previously, poor nutrition, cancer, old age, immunocompromised state, and many other conditions can slow the healing process.

The process of healing any wound has several stages. The first is hemostasis. Bleeding into the wound activates the body's clotting mechanisms. Wounds that are actively bleeding cannot heal.

The next stage is the inflammatory stage. Even the simplest wound, a paper cut, for example, initiates a cascade of biochemical and cellular responses that start the healing process. White blood cells go to work ingesting any foreign materials and fighting off bacteria. A number of inflammatory and immunologic processes lay the groundwork for the next stages of healing which are collagen deposition, angiogenesis, and myofibroblastic migration. These processes lay the structural foundation for healing, stimulate the ingrowth of new blood vessels, and promote contraction of the wound, decreasing its size. Ultimately, remodeling occurs which eventually leads to the formation of a mature scar.

Impairment of the complex wound healing process opens the door to infection and, conversely, established infection can inhibit wound healing. Patients with underlying conditions that make them at risk for poor healing require greater vigilance in the post operative period and may necessitate alterations in surgical technique or procedure to compensate for their impairment.

For example, a frail elderly patient undergoing an emergency surgery for a perforated colon needs some modifications that anticipate potential complications. Suspected poor nutrition coupled with the active infection and peritonitis that accompany perforations of the intestine should lead to changes in technique, such as closing the abdomen with large retention sutures, leaving the skin open, possibly leaving the patient on a ventilator; all maneuvers designed to anticipate and mitigate potential complications. These complications are primarily infectious, caused by our familiar villain, bacteria, that could take the opportunity to thrive in such a patient, overwhelm him, and lead to his demise.

Poor wound healing leads to infection in number of ways. Most obvious is the breakdown of wounds and repairs. An intestinal anastamosis, that is, intestine that has been reconnected after a portion has been removed, that fails to heal allows the resident bacteria to escape into the peritoneal cavity, establishing an infection secondary to a fistula. A fistula is a hole in an organ that allows its contents to escape into a surrounding area, causing an abscess, an abnormal connection to an adjacent organ or drainage through the skin and out of the body. These fistulae may heal spontaneously or may require a second, (or third or fourth), surgery to repair.

The most common example of poor healing is the breakdown of a skin wound either caused by infection or leading to infection. The wound that has failed to heal often needs to be left open and allowed to heal by what's called secondary intention, often over several weeks or even months. Such open wounds are invariably colonized by bacteria, similar to our skin, but will heal as long as the number of bacteria is not overwhelming. The open wound gradually develops a pink, granular hue, then turns a deeper shade of red as angiogenesis stimulates the growth of new blood vessels and then new skin grows in from the edges; a process called epithelialization.

Surgery requires that the villain and his accomplices be kept at bay. Absolute aseptic technique, hemostasis and proper judgment in choosing the appropriate operation in light of the patient's overall condition, as well as ensuring that conditions are maintained that promote satisfactory wound healing are all essential components of a successful operation. However, even in the most ideal of situations the outcome can be less than perfect. It is one of the realities surgeons face, a consequence of operating on the remarkable, but imperfect human machine.

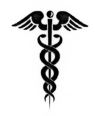

10. *The Middle of the Night*

You never have to change anything you got up in the middle of the night to write."

—Saul Bellow

Humans are constructed in remarkable and amazing ways, but, despite the incredible design things still malfunction. That is why there are doctors. It would be nice if people would have the consideration to only get sick between the hours of eight and five. Unfortunately, heart attacks, appendicitis, gall bladder attacks, strokes, and every other malady cannot tell time. They strike at any and every hour and, in the process, upset the orderly lives of everyone involved. Besides the patient and friends and family, this usually involves a doctor, along with other healthcare personnel.

When patients get sick at odd hours their options are limited. If they have an established relationship with a doctor the first step is usually a phone call. A tired voice at the answering service or the doctor's own, more modern answering system, will state: "If this is a life threatening emergency, please hang up and dial 911 or go to the nearest Emergency Room." It is unclear how the caller is to determine it is a life threatening emergency unless the opportunity to speak with a doctor or nurse is available. Still, suppose this patient has navigated the maze of options and has found himself in the local Emergency Room at two a.m., triage has been performed, tests have been ordered, and there has been actual contact with the ER physician who has told the patient that the CT Scan of his abdomen suggests a perforated duodenal ulcer and a surgeon is on the way. The patient thinks a million different thoughts, all of them ending up in a morgue, while waiting for the surgeon to arrive.

Meanwhile, at the surgeon's home, the phone rings, or chimes, or plays the Hallelujah Chorus and the surgeon is roused from a sound sleep or is interrupted, no matter what is going on at the time. The ER physician goes through his story and finally states that the CT Scan reveals free intraperitoneal air and they think it's due to a perforated ulcer, a true emergency. The surgeon jumps, or crawls, or slides out of bed, makes a quick stop in the bathroom, and heads to the hospital. The patient is interviewed, examined, appropriate personnel are called, orders written, and the patient is trundled off to the OR where anesthesia is induced, the hole is found, sutured closed with four stitches, patched with omentum, the abdomen closed and the patient goes to the recovery room, then spends 4-5 days in the hospital after which he is discharged home for a few more weeks convalescence before being declared "well" and normal activity is resumed.

The sick patient is the center of that scenario; but it is a scenario that may be repeated, in various forms, night after night. For doctors and especially for surgeons, getting up in the middle of the night is a reality that they learn to live with starting in medical school. The smart doctors go into dermatology or radiology or something similar, all very important, but also free of troublesome, life-threatening, middle-of-the-night emergencies.

So, how does the surgeon cope? Of course, it is unusual in this day and age for a surgeon to be on call night after night. Coverage is rotated between members of the group or surgeons on staff at the hospital. For myself, I have had times when I have been up for most of three days and nights. Early on in my training days I learned to grab a few minutes rest when I could. Lying down for fifteen minutes, even without sleep, does wonders. And, our bodies are equipped with adrenal glands, wonderful organs that crank up the machinery in times of stress. In all the years I've been practicing I cannot recall a single instance where a patient's care was compromised because I was tired.

However, there was at least one instance when I knew I was too tired to do surgery properly. I had been on call on a Wednesday, was up all night, and then ended up working very late into the night on Thursday. I was supposed to be on call Friday, also. When Friday rolled around I was still dead tired. I notified one of my partners who graciously covered for me.

Experience also is a great ally. When I began my career I frequently made the trek into the hospital at night; doing appendectomies, evaluating patients with belly pain, seeing any post op patients that weren't recovering as smoothly as expected. However, as the years have passed I've learned a bit of discernment. The immense improvements in diagnostic testing, coupled with confidence in my ability to decipher true emergencies, ones that require immediate attention from the urgent situations that can wait a few hours, has allowed me to avoid many unnecessary trips to the hospital. I can't recall any patients that suffered any ill effects. Most patients with appendicitis can wait a few hours with no ill effects; even truer for gallbladder attacks and most diverticulitis. But, there are some conditions that mandate expeditious intervention. Ruptured abdominal aortic aneurysms, acute arterial occlusions involving major arteries, gangrene, or perforation of the bowel all require immediate evaluation and, usually, emergency surgery. Patients whose diagnosis is not clear and who are not completely stable also warrant a middle of the night visit. Post operative patients that a nurse calls about, out of concern that something may be seriously amiss, also should be seen in person. In short, any call about a patient that leaves me wondering about their true condition will cause me to get out of bed and drive to the hospital so that I can evaluate them in person. Over the years I've learned that if I don't make the trip, I will lie awake in bed and think about it until I get up, drive to the hospital and assure myself that everything is OK. The peace of mind from seeing things in person is far preferable to hours of worry and usually of great benefit to a sick patient.

My wife has always been amazed that I have never grumbled about such middle of the night excursions and I guess that's true. Years ago I decided that middle of the night intrusions to attend to true emergencies are necessary, so it's best to just accept them and do what's right. There's always time to sleep later. And, if a doctor just can't function unless he gets seven or eight hours of uninterrupted sleep every night, then surgery is the wrong line of work.

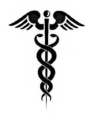

11. Decisions

Good decisions come from experience, and experience comes from bad decisions.

—Author Unknown

From the first contact with a new patient to the final post operative visit and even into the future every surgery requires a series of decisions. Should the patient undergo an operation, what is the best procedure for this particular patient with this particular problem, when should the surgery be done, what approach is best, does the patient need further evaluation or preparation, is there a serious post operative complication, and on and on. The education of a surgeon is designed to teach him or her to face each decision with the proper knowledge and confidence necessary to successfully carry the patient through the procedure and to return him or her to a full and normal life.

When I was growing up I spent a great deal of time at the race track. In high school, betting on horse races was one of the few ways I knew where I could actually profit from being smart. The art of "picking winners" involves studying the past performances of each contestant and, based on this database, picking the single horse that appears ready to win. When I started in medicine I soon learned that my years of handicapping horse races uniquely prepared me for being a doctor. After all, what is making a diagnosis and establishing a treatment plan, but picking the winner from a long list of possible maladies that could be affecting an individual, then backing up the choice with the prescribing of a medication or an act of surgery?

The decision making process begins with the history and physical, then reviewing any x-ray or lab data to establish the appropriate diagnosis. If further testing is necessary to improve the decision-making process, it is usually ordered at this time. After all the information has been gathered, the first big decision is made. Treatment options are discussed and the patient and surgeon reach agreement on a plan; be it surgery, non-operative treatment with medication, or, in some cases, no treatment. Often, one would assume the decision-making process is straightforward, certain conditions require a certain intervention, such as in the case of a patient with free intraperitoneal air. Free intraperitoneal air is a condition that is caused 99.99% of the time by the perforation of a hollow organ, that is, stomach or intestine.

However, this one-time universal indication for immediate emergency surgery is no longer quite so universal. In these days of improved imaging with very sensitive CT Scanners it is common to encounter patients with clinical symptoms of diverticulitis, which is infection around the colon secondary to an inflamed or ruptured diverticulum. Such diverticuli are weak areas of the colon that balloon out between the fibers of the outer muscular layer and are very common cause of hospitalization. Before highly sensitive CT scanners were the norm, diagnosis and treatment were based on the clinical findings coupled with plain x-rays and blood tests. If a patient demonstrated "free" air on a plain abdominal or chest x-ray immediate emergency surgery was performed and, if the perforation was secondary to diverticular disease, they would usually end up with a temporary colostomy.

In today's modern world it is very common to see tiny bubbles of "free" air on CT scans in a patient who clinically seems to have uncomplicated diverticulitis. So the cut and dry decision-making process is muddled and the surgeon has to consider all the possibilities to make a decision. Is this patient likely to recover with a non operative approach or is immediate surgery still the best option? Is there middle ground, temporizing measure that would be best. Cookbook medicine won't work in such situations. Indeed, there are few situations where the cookbook approach ever works.

So, the decision-making process is very similar to handicapping a horse race. Look at all the available data, weigh each factor appropriately and put your money down. Ten dollars to win on appendicitis. In the end we surgeons hope the winner is the patient.

Consider appendicitis: a common surgical problem whose diagnosis is made even easier in these modern days with modern imaging. A sixteen-year-old male comes to the ER with 24-hour history of abdominal pain localized to the right lower quadrant of the abdomen, low grade fever, a little nausea, elevated white blood count, localized signs of peritonitis, and a CT scan that reveals a dilated, thickened appendix. It's 3:00 a.m. There's no question of the diagnosis or the appropriate treatment; only one question remains: Should I do the surgery now or wait until the next day? The decision in this case is probably not based on the patient's clinical condition, rather it becomes a scheduling issue. Is the OR very busy the next day? Is the surgeon's schedule the next day busy? The reality is that such issues are often important in a case like this.

But, let's make a few changes. The same sixteen-year-old male presents with the same symptoms, only now the CT scan reveals a dilated, fluid-filled appendix. This one fact should change the decision-making process. Such a finding suggests that this appendix is more likely to rupture and cause generalized peritonitis or an abscess. In this situation it is in the patient's best interest to do the surgery immediately.

Now, suppose another change is made. The same patient presents with the same symptoms, except the CT scan is normal. Should the surgeon follow his clinical judgment and remove the appendix, which is reported as normal on the CT scan, or send the patient home (unlikely), or admit the patient and observe him for a period of time? Or, suppose the patient has only had pain for 12 hours, but still has clinical findings suggestive of appendicitis and a normal CT scan.

My answer would be to operate on the latter patient and observe the former. 12 hours may not be enough time for inflammation to appear on a CT scan; a patient with all the clinical findings suggestive of appendicitis for such a short time warrants surgery. However, twenty four hours should be adequate time for some inflammation to appear on the scan and it then becomes more likely that the abdominal pain is caused by a condition other than appendicitis. In either case a surgeon would not be faulted for either proceeding with surgery or observation in the hospital for a period of time.

But, suppose another variable is changed. Instead of a sixteen-year-old boy, the patient is an 86-year-old male and the CT Scan reveals inflammation in the area of the appendix, but the appendix itself is not visualized. Add another kicker, the patient is anemic with a hemoglobin of nine (anemia is a low blood count; the normal hemoglobin level in a male is around fourteen). The possibilities increase. An elderly patient is more likely to have other medical conditions. Anemia is commonly caused by occult blood loss associated with colon cancer, particularly in the right colon. Ischemia of the colon often affects the cecum, this portion of the colon being most distant from the origin of the superior mesenteric artery, which is the principal arterial supply, making the ileocolic bowel most vulnerable to low perfusion states that can be associated with congestive heart failure, a condition common to the elderly, but extremely rare in a sixteen year old.

So the horse race becomes more competitive and selecting a winner requires more study. Now suppose our patient is female. Even the sixteen-year-old can become a challenge. Young men with appendicitis usually do not present a great diagnostic challenge. But women have Fallopian tubes, ovaries, and uteri. They can get pregnant or have endometriosis. In the ancient pre-CT scan days, thirty years ago, most of the negative appendectomies were in women of child bearing age. Even with scanning the diagnosis may not be clear. Watchful waiting is always a useful adjunct and it is at such times a CT scan is helpful. Even if the diagnosis is unclear; sometimes the scan will suggest it's time to take a look and sometimes it will say it's OK to wait. Judgment, knowledge, experience and a little horse sense all play a role in the decision-making process. In the end we surgeons always hope we've backed the right horse.

II. Intraoperative

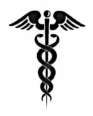

12. Barriers

To me the ideal doctor would be a man endowed with profound knowledge of life and of the soul, intuitively divining any suffering or disorder of whatever kind, and restoring peace by his mere presence.

—Henri Amiel

In the practice of surgery it is necessary to create barriers; obstacles that separate the surgeon from his patient. During any operation the surgeon and his assistants wear gowns, caps, masks, and gloves which act as a barrier between the patient and the OR crew. These protective items help prevent contamination of the surgical field; keeping the bacteria that reside on our skin and in our mouths and noses from infecting the surgical wound. Indeed, certain orthopedic procedures, those in which any introduction of bacteria can be a life threatening disaster, take this barrier precaution to the extreme. The orthopedist has adopted an elaborate system of helmets and filters, strictly limits access to the room during the procedure and does everything humanly possible to banish the potentially deadly microorganism from the OR suite.

There is, however, much more to the barrier concept than protection of the patient. Unfortunately, it is a necessity of modern times that the OR crew also be protected; protected from contamination by the patient. It is one of the sad facts of our modern world that chronic infectious diseases exist. It is an almost daily occurrence that medical personnel will be called upon to care for patients with HIV, hepatitis B or C, MRSA, and a host of other infectious agents that have the potential to be transmissible from the patient to OR personnel during the course of an operation. Proper barriers, proper technique, and appropriate choice of operation protect us from our own patients and allow us the opportunity to live and serve another day.

At the end of most operations the final mechanical barrier is left with the patient, the surgical dressing. I have seen such dressings raised to the level of ritual, the surgeon mandating that only certain materials placed in a certain way be used, instructing the patient to leave the dressing in place for exactly 76 hours and 12 minutes and then remove it at precisely the proper time, unless there is a full moon, in which case it needs to be left until dawn the following day. A bit of an exaggeration, surely, but not as much as you might think. Personally, I think that a simple dressing is best; something that can be removed easily and painlessly in 48 hours.

The surgical dressing certainly is important, particularly for the first few hours. Most surgical wounds, however, are probably sealed from the outside world within twenty four hours. As a matter of fact, I instruct my hemorrhoidectomy patients to remove their dressings after only about six hours; for comfort and to begin proper care of the area. It is an extremely rare event for these patients to develop an infection, surprising really, given the location and environment of such surgery. There are reasons why infections in this area are rare which involve an entirely different sort of biological barrier, but that is a subject for another article.

There is another type of barrier that is necessarily built up between patient and physician. This is the psychological barrier; an invisible wall that prevents excessive bonding between a doctor and his patient, thus preserving an appropriate doctor-patient relationship, one that is intimate on a medically therapeutic level only. Medical School, at least my medical school, taught us to maintain an aloof concern for our patients, supposedly for the patient's well being and to maintain our objectivity.

An excessively close relationship can make the patient too reliant on their doctor, while at the same time potentially cloud the physician's judgment, leading to decisions based upon feelings, rather than proper objective findings. I carry this concept to its extreme in my novel, *Joshua and Aaron,* as the doctors are prohibited from actually examining the patients in person. Such a scenario is unlikely, you are thinking, but the trend is already present.

Today, a patient visiting an emergency room is initially seen by a triage nurse, who makes the initial assessment of the severity of the condition and very often orders the indicated tests to help establish a diagnosis. After such tests are completed the emergency room physician will finally see the patient and confirm a diagnosis that has already been established. It won't be long until the doctor becomes a superfluous intermediary and is completely eliminated from the equation. (Obamacare here we come.)

It's not just in emergency rooms such a scene plays out. The pressures of modern medicine force doctors to spend less and less time with the patient as regulations, paperwork and diminishing reimbursement force the doctor to do more and more in a limited period of time. However, don't think that the quality of care suffers in such a system, because this definitely is not true. The amazing array of imaging systems and lab tests has made medical diagnosis far more accurate now than it was thirty years ago. What is lost is the personal aspect, the unique doctor-patient relationship that makes a doctor an ally, advocate, and friend.

In my surgical practice we have a physician's assistant, whose job is to assist us in the operating room. When she first started with us, our office manager asked me if I wanted her to help in the office. My answer was no. Surgery today requires much shorter hospital stays and the contact between surgeon and patient is greatly limited. Generally, I will see my patient once in the office; surgery will be scheduled, they'll be seen again immediately before the operation and then once or twice more in the office afterwards. This is a far cry from years ago when the patient, for a similar operation, would go into the hospital the day before surgery and then stay for one or two weeks afterwards. All this personal contact certainly strengthened the physician patient relationship and lowered the barriers that existed, but in no way did it actually improve patient care or final outcome.

The current system is more economical and far better for the patient. But, it throws up a barrier of sorts. That is why I refused to have our PA see patients in the office. I am given one chance to create a relationship with my patient before surgery and I do not want anything or anyone to diminish this already limited opportunity.

There is one particular medical condition where I do everything possible to break down the barrier that exists between doctor and patient and that is with breast cancer patients. Of course all patients are important and most every type of cancer is serious, but of all the different diseases I encounter this one creates the greatest emotions and intense feelings for the patient and family and perhaps for the treating physician. I am often the physician called upon to inform a woman (99% of the time it's a woman) of the diagnosis of breast cancer. Usually I'm the one that has performed the biopsy and often the first therapeutic intervention requires surgery. So, I have to break the news. Most of the time I've started to prepare my patient for such bad news even before the biopsy is done.

Probably 98% percent of the time when a woman comes to me with a lump in her breast or an abnormal mammogram or ultrasound it is immediately apparent whether or not the lump is cancerous. At this point I will tell her and her family that the findings are very worrisome for cancer, but that a biopsy is necessary. When I receive the confirmatory biopsy report I always tell her in person and make sure that I am not rushed for time while I explain all the implications and options. After the first explanation I usually explain everything a second and usually a third time, hoping that some of what I say will actually be retained. Even with all this many women hear nothing beyond the two words "breast cancer." It is very common to get a call a few hours later or the next day asking about all the options again.

In situations like these I do my best to tear down the invisible barrier that exists between doctor and patient. The trust that is built in those moments contributes tremendously to healing for the patient and their family. It isn't bad for the doctor, either.

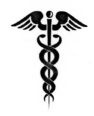

13. Seconds, Minutes, Hours

To think too long about doing a thing often becomes its undoing.

—Eva Young

Sometimes in the practice of surgery it is necessary to work very quickly. The ABC's of trauma stand for "Airway, Breathing, Circulation" and management of problems in each of these areas often requires that a procedure be done very fast. A patient's life usually depends on it.

In the management of trauma, but also any emergency, airway is always the primary consideration. If there is no airway, the patient dies. Most of the time airways are secured by endotracheal intubation, a fancy expression that means passing a tube through the mouth or nose into the trachea to maintain a passage for breathing or assisting the patient with breathing. But, what if the tube can't be passed the usual way? The mouth or nose is blocked by swelling or blood or injuries; such a crisis calls for somebody, most always a surgeon, to open an airway, usually by cutting a hole directly through the neck.

Seconds count and a sharp scalpel is really important. Over the years I've had to act in such situations perhaps a dozen times. The most unforgettable was a five-year-old girl who had been in a motor vehicle accident, a very serious one that killed both her parents and also injured her brother. She arrived at our ER, unstable, no IV, no airway, barely alive. A very experienced and adept anesthetist did his best to intubate her, while my most competent senior resident established IV access. It soon became apparent that she could not be intubated in the usual manner. Fortunately, she had a thin neck and at that moment I grabbed the scalpel that had been used to cut down on her saphenous vein, quickly felt the landmarks on her neck, and started to cut. In less than thirty seconds I had created an opening in her cricothyroid membrane; the anesthetist gave me an appropriate size tube which I managed to slide through the hole and down into her trachea so she could be ventilated. Unfortunately, her injuries were very severe, involving both chest and abdomen, as well as a severe intracranial injury and she only survived few hours.

I had a similar situation about a year later. Now an attending, instead of Chief Resident, I had just finished assisting the Chief Resident on the Vascular service with the repair of a ruptured abdominal aortic aneurysm; successfully, at least up to the point where the patient was transferred to the ICU. While the Chief Resident was talking to the family I waited in the ICU. The patient was very swollen from head to toe, typical after such a surgery where the patient requires large volumes of fluids and multiple transfusions. He seemed to be properly settled in the ICU as the radiology technicians wheeled their portable x-ray machine in to take a routine post op chest x-ray. This x-ray required lifting the patients back to slide the film plate under his back. During this process, the patient's endotracheal tube became entangled with the ventilator tubes and supports and in a single, dire moment the tube slid out, leaving this very swollen, almost completely anesthetized patient without an airway and not breathing.

The anesthesia team was still at hand, but they couldn't even see the back of his throat. A tracheostomy tray, always on hand in this particular ICU, was cracked open and I started to cut into his thick, short neck. This time there were no landmarks, everything obscured by the swollen tissue. But, in times of need sometimes you get lucky. I actually came right down on his trachea and managed to pop a tube in; the entire ordeal taking about two minutes. This patient fared only a bit better, surviving for about two weeks, before succumbing to a combination of kidney and respiratory failure.

After "A" for airway issues, breathing is the "B" in ABC. Fortunately, in a hospital setting, assuming the role of breathing for the sick and injured is rarely a problem. "Ambu" bags and oxygen are almost always readily available. But, what if they're available, but a mechanical ventilator is not? In this situation, some poor unfortunate individual, hopefully with strong hands, has to stand at the patients head and squeeze the "Ambu" bag steadily until the patient can breathe on his own or a ventilator is connected or something else happens to make such ventilation unnecessary.

Years ago, in Houston, tropical storm Alison blew through, flooding the streets of the city and also flooding many of the downtown buildings. In particular, Hermann Hospital's basement was flooded, ruining millions of dollars of research, but, also, knocking out all the power to the hospital. Patients that were dependent on mechanical ventilation now had to be "bagged," meaning someone had to stand by and manually squeeze the "Ambu," assuming the role of breathing for that patient. At the same time all these patients needed to be evacuated from the powerless building. So, there was a procession of critically ill patients being carefully ferried down stairwells, illumination provided by a few emergency lights and flashlights, in sweltering early summer Houston heat, each patient attended by nurses, residents and interns; with one unlucky intern given the task of ventilating the patient. It isn't known if any patient died during this time, but all the hospital staff were heroes.

Finally, there is "C," circulation; the restoration and maintenance of adequate blood flow. Patients that are bleeding or have compromise of circulation for other reasons usually are in the state called "shock," manifested by low blood pressure, rapid heart rate, and poor organ perfusion, all of which lead to altered sensorium, decreased urine output, and ultimately organ failure and death.

Patients in shock require rapid intervention to restore adequate circulation. Often, the treatment can be as simple as administering intravenous fluids or blood. But, while this resuscitation is ongoing the cause must also be addressed. Bleeding, heart failure and severe infection are common and such sources must be identified and treated.

Bleeding, for example, is the most common cause of shock in the injured patient. Guns, knives and car accidents have a way of cutting, tearing, and mangling blood vessels and organs which cause bleeding, sometimes massively. At these times, it is necessary to work quickly and efficiently. Trauma surgeons speak of the "Golden Hour" which is the first hour after injury. The goal is to resuscitate, diagnose, and begin to treat the life and limb threatening injuries in this first hour.

Major blood vessels in the neck, chest, abdomen, or extremities can bleed profusely when injured and control of such injuries is essential if the injured patient is to be saved. In this day and age diagnosis is usually expeditious. Treatment almost always means surgery and time matters. The quicker the bleeding source can be identified and controlled the better the outcome. Still the body does provide mechanisms that buy a little time. Luckily for all surgeons, blood clots and, especially for major arteries, vessels constrict. This is why a patient that has severed his arm doesn't bleed to death, a vessel cut cleanly through certainly bleeds for a while, but as the blood pressure falls, the vessel narrows and a clot will form on the end. This buys the surgeon crucial minutes to get control of the situation and allows for an orderly repair. However, an artery cut lengthwise is a bit problematical, is more likely to continue to bleed and can be the cause of exsanguinations.

Such was the case years ago, when I was seeing far more trauma patients. A young man was brought into the Emergency Room with severe hypotension. He had been burglarizing a home and broke a window to gain entrance. In the process he must have caught his right arm on a sharp edge of glass. The police reported massive amounts of blood at the crime scene, almost as if the thief thought the spray of blood was amusing. The patient suffered cardiac arrest almost the moment he came through the door and, despite all efforts, he could not be saved. The only injury that could be found was a deep, linear laceration on his upper arm, over his brachial artery, the main artery that carries blood to the arm and hand.

Sometimes, all efforts are for naught. Massive blood loss uses up clotting factors, massive transfusion results in a cold, washed out patient whose blood won't clot; even if the major vessels have been repaired, all the small unnamed capillaries and arterioles can continue a relentless oozing of blood that is every bit as massive as would be expected from the aorta. In such a situation there are few options, pack gauze sponges everywhere to tamponade the bleeding until the underlying clotting problem and hypothermia are corrected. This goes beyond seconds and minutes, often taking hours or days and creates new, different problems: infection, organ dysfunction, common causes of patient demise in such situations.

So, when pressed a surgeon needs to work quickly, do his or her best to repair the injured party, minimize the consequences of injury, and, hopefully, see the patient live to walk-out of the hospital.

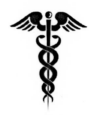

14. Trust

Few things help an individual more than to place responsibility upon him, and to let him know that you trust him.

—Booker T. Washington

The hallmark of the medical profession is trust. Consider that from start to finish every aspect of patient care depends on trust. The patient trusts his or her doctor to do what is in their best interest, prescribe the proper medication, order the most appropriate tests, and, when necessary, refer to a specialist that will provide expert and compassionate care.

In surgery this trust extends even farther. The patient literally places every aspect of their being into the hands of the doctors, nurses, and technicians that are performing the operation. From the instrument technician, to the patient aid that transports the patient to the OR, the surgical team works together to provide the utmost, skilled care to an individual that is probably frightened, worried, and, perhaps, thinking that their life is near its end. At such a time the patient places all his trust in the crew.

The trust does not stop with the patient, however. I was thinking about this the other day as the surgical tech was handing me a scalpel. Just like on television, I held out my hand and the razor sharp instrument appeared, properly oriented and ready to be used. All done without the need for me to even look up or watch what was being done. Then, through the course of the surgery all I had to do was put out my hand, mumble an unintelligible word, and the proper instrument magically appeared. Such well coordinated events don't always occur, but an experienced tech can be trusted to make the operation run smoothly and quickly.

But what of the rest of the team? I trust the floor nurse to have all the pre-op medications given, to help allay any fears the patient may have had and, often, call me if something isn't quite right, to express concerns that perhaps the patient isn't ready.

The pre-op nurse checks everything once again, insures that the patient is aware of what is being done and that everyone agrees on the proposed procedure. In the actual OR suite the circulating nurse helps position the patient, often assists the anesthesiologist with the induction, and then does the final preparation before the start of surgery. During the course of the procedure, the circulator is called upon to run and get any equipment that may not already be in the room, anticipating the needs of the surgical technician and the surgeon.

The anesthesiologist literally has every aspect of the patient's life in his hands. The art and science of anesthesia has come a long way from the infant days of ether and nitrous oxide. The great improvement in perioperative and intraoperative monitoring have made general anesthesia very safe and effective. The anesthesiologist now can have continuous monitoring of cardiac, neurologic, pulmonary, renal and metabolic activity; all while never taking his eyes off the Wall

Street Journal (just kidding). Continuous EKG, pulse oximetry, BIS monitors and a host of other devices allow the patient to place complete trust in his anesthesiologist.

After the surgery intensive monitoring continues under the watchful eye of the PACU (recovery room) nurse. During the crucial first hour after any surgery that required general anesthesia, the PACU nurse sits with the patient ready to intervene with a jaw thrust or ambu bag should any ill effects from the surgery or anesthesia develop. Fortunately, 99% of the time all that is necessary is expectant observation, followed by transport and hand-off to the last member of the OR crew. The nurse in the day surgery unit or on the post surgical floor helps the patient through the later recovery phase of any operation until the time of discharge.

There are many others involved in the successful completion of a surgical procedure. Respiratory therapists, physical therapists, occupational therapists, technicians from many different departments, as well as physicians of every specialty all play a role in the care of the surgical patient and all have earned the trust of the surgical staff.

But, what if trust is lost or absent? Would it be possible for me to do my job properly and expeditiously if trust was lacking? Of course, the surgery could be done and, most likely, without too much fuss. But a lack of trust between any members of the surgical crew raises stress levels and the potential for complications rises. Unfortunately, I have seen situations where the anesthesiologist or circulating nurse expressed a sense of dread at having to do a particular case with a particular surgeon. They don't trust the surgeon to do the job in a way that minimizes stress or in an expeditious manner. Dreading a particular surgeon or procedure is a bad way for the OR team to commence. Similarly, I have to say that that there have been times when I have not trusted a particular anesthesiologist to do a particular surgery. This situation arose much more in the past, when the variability between the different anesthesia personnel was more pronounced. Complicated surgery on patients with multiple comorbidities calls for the highest level of intraoperative care and monitoring. There have been times when I have cancelled or postponed an operation, rather than allow my patient to receive potentially substandard care. Happily, this hasn't happened in years, as all the anesthesia personnel in the facilities I work provide excellent care.

An operation is dependent on trust from start to finish. If such trust does not exist or is lost, the entire process becomes suspect and the outcome and the patient suffer.

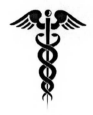

15. Under Tension

Tension is who you think you should be. Relaxation is who you are.

—Chinese Proverb

The actual performance of surgery involves a great deal of tension. This tension, however, is not the type of tension, you might expect. The perception that the surgeon is under a great deal of tension is usually not true. The training of the surgeon involves gradually increasing responsibility, designed to eliminate any undue tension or stress. No, the tension I'm talking about is the type that is necessary to perform an operation properly.

In medical school there was a gruff general surgeon named Dr. Adams. He terrorized residents and medical students with his loud and crusty demeanor, but really had a heart of gold. His primary purpose was to produce physicians, surgeons in particular, who would execute their duties with the greatest care and skill. One of his mantras was "tissue under tension." Anyone practicing the art of surgery knows that this saying is central to any surgical procedure.

Tissue under tension allows proper dissection; but also can lead to post operative disaster.

One of the little secrets of surgical technique is that actually doing an operation usually is not that difficult. God, in His infinite wisdom, has equipped many parts of His creation with white lines that tell the surgeon exactly where to place his scalpel or scissors and where it is safe to cut. Thus, during a colon resection, for example, the surgeon dissects along these clearly marked tissue planes and stays away from areas that are potentially troubling.

This is where tension comes in. Retraction of the tissues being dissected reveals these "dotted lines" that say "cut here." Such lines of dissection remain obscure if proper tension is not applied. Too much tension may create false planes of dissection and lead to unwanted organ injury. So, the art of surgery is really one of proper exposure and application of tension. The really great technical surgeons usually come by this skill naturally and most surgical educators recognize when one of their residents demonstrates such talent.

However, this skill can be learned and great surgeons can also be made. Any surgeon that takes the time to perform an operation carefully and with proper attention to detail will be successful. Following the mantra of "tissue under tension" is one way to become a technically skilled surgeon. The surgeon that rushes through a procedure, ignores all the basic rules and takes unnecessary and potentially dangerous "shortcuts" is the one that ends up with complications. Such attempts to cut corners almost always end up costing more for the patient and the surgeon, taking more time and resources in the long run.

So, tension is important during surgical dissection. The other end of the spectrum is reconstruction after the dissection, resection or excision is complete. For instance, after resecting a cancerous segment of colon it is always necessary to reconstruct the gastrointestinal tract in some manner. This usually involves connecting one divided end of intestine to another. In this situation tension is bad. Dr. Adams' mantra is truly a double edged sword.

Intestinal anastamosis, (reconnection), under excessive tension leads to disaster. Improper healing with subsequent breakdown of the anastamosis results in a very sick or dead patient. Tension is one of the primary causes of such an occurrence.

When tissue is brought together under tension; stretched beyond acceptable limits, it may appear to the naked eye to be perfectly fine. But such tension stretches and narrows the blood vessels supplying these tissues. This compromised vascular supply, be it veins, arteries, or both, can lead to poor healing. Taking the time to adequately mobilize and dissect the organs necessary for reconstruction, avoiding any tension that may inhibit the healing process is one of the hallmarks of a skilled technical surgeon.

However, there are times when excessive tissue tension is deliberately employed. In the arena of the plastic surgeon "tissue under tension" intentionally comes into play. When people think of plastic surgery their first thoughts are of face lifts, breast implants and nose jobs. But, what the Plastic surgery really does is stretch the limits of the tissues. Thus, a facelift stretches the skin of the face to achieve an excellent cosmetic result, all the while taking care to preserve an adequate blood and nerve supply.

The reconstructive aspect of plastic surgery takes this even farther. Skin flaps and muscle flaps move tissues on a pedicle of blood supply, artery and vein, to an adjacent area that needs new tissue. Reconstructing breasts and faces after cancer surgery, rebuilding tissues damaged by radiation therapy, and similar procedures extend the tissue under tension creed to the limit. Occasionally, the limits may necessarily be exceeded which led to the use of surgical leeches.

We are all aware of leeches, bloodsucking animals that have no purpose except to gorge themselves on the blood of unsuspecting men and beasts until they fall off, fat and happy. Who would think that these parasites have a therapeutic purpose? Surprisingly, they do. In some situations, primarily reimplantation of severed appendages, the replanted organ can become engorged with blood. Veins that were reconnected may become swollen and not function properly for several days. Coming to the rescue, like a heroic white knight, is the medical grade leech. They don't require any special training; they just do what comes naturally. Latch them on to the vulnerable finger or ear and they go to work, greedily stuffing themselves with the patient's blood and, at the same time, preventing vascular engorgement that would lead to gangrene. These remarkable creatures have their own anticoagulant that prevents unwanted clotting and when they are full, they simply fall off signaling to the nurse or doctor to get a new one.

It is apparent that tension in the operating room is integral to the success of almost any surgery. The surgeon learns to utilize tension when it is beneficial and avoid it when it is detrimental. And, at all times, he tries to eliminate psychological tension. One of the truisms of surgery is that procedures that are common, mundane, and boring are always preferred. Interesting cases are fun to read about, but boring is better. This does not mean that the routine, common operations receive any less care or consideration. Every case is treated with the utmost attention to detail and concern. But, difficult surgery on very sick patients can create an atmosphere of tension. One of the distinguishing features of an experienced and well trained surgeon is that there are very few situations where psychological tension is allowed to rear its ugly head during the course of an operation. Shouting, throwing instruments and other inappropriate behavior by operating room staff creates an atmosphere of stress and tension that focuses attention away from the patient and contributes to poorer outcomes. Even during the most difficult operations, cool hands and cool heads should prevail and tension should be relegated to the tissues being dissected.

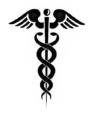

16. Hands

As you grow older, you will discover that you have two hands, one for helping yourself, the other for helping others.

—Audrey Hepburn

What does a surgeon do exactly? How can a surgeon tell that this organ is diseased, that one is the source of this patient's problem, this other appears abnormal only because it is reacting in response to another issue? How does a surgeon know where to cut and why doesn't the patient bleed to death from the skin incision? When I was younger these are questions I asked myself and it wasn't until I was into my residency that they were all answered. Of course bleeding has been discussed elsewhere (see "Accomplices"), but the other questions are at the heart of surgical technique.

The good from the bad, the determination is usually not very hard. Normal tissue is soft and pliable. Even solid organs, like the liver, spleen, and kidneys feel smooth and soft in their normal state. In the early days of modern surgery,

William Halsted eschewed his newly invented rubber gloves, rather than give up the improved tactile sense of bare hands. Gradually, sterility won out and he grudgingly donned the rubber gloves. Of course, gloves have improved and we now have "Sensors" and "Super Sensitive" gloves and surgeons quickly learn how to "feel" while wearing sterile gloves. But, what do they feel?

When disease strikes, be it infection, cancer, or inflammation, the tissue becomes hard and stiff. Cancer almost always feels hard and almost always stands out from adjacent, normal tissue. An inflamed appendix feels hard compared to a normal one. When an abdominal operation is done for cancer or appendicitis or for most diseases, the first thing a surgeon will do is run his hand over all the viscera to feel where the offending organ is hiding. Most often the area in question is known prior to surgery and the confirmatory tactile exploration is more for the surgeon's benefit than the patient's. In a similar vein, but far coarser, many surgeons, myself included, will palpate the patient's abdomen as soon as the anesthetic induction is completed. At this time the patient is completely relaxed and this pre-incision abdominal exam is done partially for education and partially for preparation.

If an operation is being done for an acute inflammatory condition; appendicitis, cholecystitis, or diverticulitis (being most common), and a mass is easily felt through the abdominal wall of the anesthetized patient, then the surgery may turn out to be more complicated than originally anticipated. Inflammation that is significant enough to cause such a mass, which is usually composed of omentum and adjacent organs which surround and seal off the diseased area, usually means that getting to the true pathology may be a difficult and tedious process. If I can easily feel an inflamed gallbladder on abdominal palpation prior to beginning a laparoscopic cholecystectomy, I'll often warn the OR crew that the surgery may need to be open and to be prepared.

Hands, it seems, are important for finding diseased organs, but what else do our hands do? The tactile sense is often important for dissection. Get into the right tissue plane, put your finger in and the colon is soon lifted out of its usual resting place and ready to plucked out, along with any offending tumors. During operations for trauma, where speed is often most important, hand dissection can quickly move normal organs out of the way, allowing access to injured organs and blood vessels.

When a surgeon enters the abdomen to fix a ruptured abdominal aortic aneurysm and is greeted by a gush of blood. What can be done to stem the tide and save a dying patient? Blindly pass your hand through the sea of red and grab the aorta where it comes through the diaphragm and squeeze it closed. It's always there, right behind the esophagus, and the hand becomes a dam, holding the pulsing flow of blood at bay until the aorta can be controlled closer to the source of bleeding, lower down in the abdomen.

Of course operations are done with more than hands. TV and movies always show the surgical tech slapping instruments into the waiting hands of the surgeon. With such clever names as Crile, Kocher, Leahy (a few of the names for various clamps), Metzenbaum or Mayo (scissors), Richardson, Deever, or Balfour (retractors), all named for the surgeon that takes credit for its invention, instruments are extensions of the surgeon's hand. They allow assistants to help, while staying out of the way; allow the surgeon to pull and hold and dissect tissues, often more delicately and with a more confident grip than fingers would allow, while increasing the surgeon's reach.

The loss in tactile sense is compensated by the improvement in tissue handling and exposure. There is still some sense of feeling, even when it is transmitted to the hand by an instrument.

But now we have modern surgery, laparoscopic or robotic, and the hand has become even more remote from the actual surgery. Laparoscopic surgery is done through small tubes that allow access to the surgical site, utilizing very small incisions. The surgeon relies on the high definition video image and sense of touch is limited to what can be transmitted through long probes, graspers, and dissectors. Still, there is some tactile sensation, even with the long laparoscopic instruments.

The advent of completely robotic surgery removes all direct contact with the patient. The surgeon sits at a console completely separated from the patient and computerized arms dissect and reconstruct the operative field. Hands are replaced by digital arms, remotely controlled by the surgeon/operator. There is no touching, no sensation of normal or abnormal, no sense of a pulsing artery immediately behind the area of dissection. Still, the robot provides great precision; as precise as the operator sitting at his console. To me, however, something seems lost. The impersonal nature of robotic surgery takes away the special bond that develops between surgeon and patient.

From Halsted to robots, the hand is still an essential surgical tool, but who knows what the future will bring? Thirty years ago laparoscopic surgery was practically nonexistent. I wonder where we'll be thirty years from now?

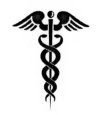

17. The Eyes and the Mind

I would like to see the day when somebody would be appointed surgeon somewhere who had no hands, for the operative part is the least part of the work.
—Harvey Cushing

That's quite a belly, rotund and smooth, the hair clipped away only moments ago. The yellow orange hew of the Chloraprep stares back at me as I pick up the scalpel and start to cut. From the xiphoid to the pubis, a long straight incision is made, with a gentle curve around the belly button; blood wells up from the skin edges and fat as I hand off the scalpel, exchanging it for the Bovie, the electrocautery device that is so essential to most of the operations I do.

The buzzing sound, followed by wisps of smoke rising up for the wound follow my trail as each individual bleeding vessel is controlled with a quick zap. This initial step completed, the incision is carried deeper. A gentle pull by me on one side and my assistant on the other, spreads the fat right down the middle and the criss cross of whitish fibers is seen, signifying the midline of the abdominal fascia, the fibrous sheath that keeps our organs from protruding out of our peritoneal cavity.

The cautery cuts through the middle exposing more fat which signifies that it is the midline, rather than either side. No muscle fibers are seen which means I've managed to stay in the middle for the entire length of the newly created wound. We elevate the tissue beneath the fascia and poke through. The space beneath immediately fills with air and the thin peritoneum lifts away from the underlying organs. More fat is seen, but this has a bit of different color, a slightly darker shade of yellow and less lobular, laced with blood vessels; my old friend, the omentum, safeguarding the other organs that lie deeper within the peritoneal cavity.

This day I have little interest in the omentum or the bowels; I delve deeper, behind all these structures. Behind the omentum and the small bowel is a potential demon, the object of today's surgery, an aortic aneurysm. As the bowels are retracted, gently packed out of my way, the bulge of the weakened artery is seen through the fat and peritoneum that separate the peritoneal cavity from the retroperitoneum. The names are very logical, providing proper order to what I hope will be a very orderly operation. Nothing unusual so far; let's hope it stays that way.

The pulsing bulge of the aortic aneurysm is obvious as the duodenum, which is the first part of the small intestine, is dissected away from the protruding, pounding mass. Quickly, the duodenum joins the rest of the bowel, out of sight and safely away from the aneurysm; the tissue over the aneurysm is divided using the cautery. Be careful, don't cut a hole in the aorta yet. The wall of the weakened blood vessel, now exposed, is followed up towards the head until it narrows back to its normal size of about 2 cm. The vessel is felt, the strong pulsations present a contrast to the, luckily, soft vessel wall.

Lucky, because it seems this aorta will be easy to sew; sometimes the aorta is rock hard with calcification in its wall, the proverbial hardening of the arteries carried to the extreme.

The tissue astride the "neck" of the aneurysm is divided, some small blood vessels clipped with titanium clips to prevent any annoying bleeding. Looks good, the neck seems long enough, there's the left renal vein, everything proceeds as orderly as possible. *Careful now, don't tear anything,* I think as I dissect along either side of the aorta down to the bones of the vertebral bodies. I grab the long, gently curved aortic clamp and ease it into position and snap it closed around the bounding, pulsing vessel. The vessel becomes quiescent, the aorta is tamed. Before the anesthesiologist can protest I unclamp the aorta and turn my attention to the rest of the dissection.

The distal aorta and the iliac arteries are exposed quickly, without incident, and a final check is made to be sure all the vessels are adequately exposed and controlled.

"How much does he weigh?" I inquire of the anesthesiologist.

"Eighty Kilos . . . give 8500 units of heparin."

Heparin is a powerful blood thinner that prevents clotting inside the aorta and other vessels while the arteries are clamped, a potential disaster should it occur. Time to wait, at least three minutes, while the heparin circulates. A good time to shift position, I move my legs and bend my knee a bit, getting rid of the tightness that always develops when I'm in a case that calls for more than the usual concentration. I take the aortic sizers and measure 20 mm. The graft always looks too small, but I've learned that the sizers are more accurate than trying to "eyeball" the aorta, at least for me.

"I'm hungry," announces my assistant from across the table. I glance at the clock, 11:00 a.m. You can set your clock by her stomach. I turn back to the surgery at hand.

Everything in readiness, proper clamps, 2-0 silk sutures loaded and ready to go; it's time. First the curved aortic clamp, slipped above the neck and pushed down to the bones behind the aorta followed by cessation of the pulsing; next, the straight clamps on the iliac arteries, then a scalpel and the aorta is punctures.

As the blood wells up out of the whole, it's all captured and sent to the "cell saver" to be washed, concentrated, and readied for return to the patient.

The weakened wall of the aorta is opened further and the lumbar arteries squirting blood through the back wall are identified and stitched closed as quickly as possible until all the bleeding has stopped. So far so good, no difficult lumbar arteries to deal with. I look at the inferior mesenteric artery; *not good,* I think. There is a dribble of blood coming back. To me it means I will need to reimplant this artery into the graft once it is in place.

If there is no blood coming back from this artery then it is already occluded, a common occurrence with aortic aneurysms, and there is no reason to reimplant it; if it is pulsing back then it can be safely tied off, the pulsatile flow indicating adequate collateral flow. So, the sluggish flow means collateral vessels may be inadequate to properly perfuse the left colon and I'll need to do a little extra work. The inferior mesenteric artery is clamped for now, to be dealt with a bit later.

Time to work and work expeditiously. This should be easy, the aorta is soft and pliable and there is enough of a cuff of normal aorta; but maybe not. The back wall seems a bit thin and the aneurysm along the back extends higher up than suggested by the pre-op scans. A twenty millimeter graft, 3-0 prolene in hand, the sewing starts. First the back wall; *please hold these sutures.* Everything seems OK; the proximal anastamosis goes quickly and in about fifteen minutes it's ready to be tested. The clamp is eased open and blood spews out from the back. The clamp is quickly closed and another 3-0 prolene finds its way into the patient. Two stitches along the back wall and another test is made. It looks good, no bleeding and a good pulse in the graft. So far, so good.

Now it's time to do the distal anastamosis. The aorta just above the bifurcation is adequate, fairly soft, not aneurismal, and the iliacs are also OK. The graft is quickly tailored to conform to the distal aorta and, with 3-0 prolene in hand the graft is sewn into place with minimal fuss. Smooth as silk, clamp time of just under one hour; it looks like we'll finish the case uneventfully. Unclamp the right leg; good pulse, no bleeding; now the left leg; no bleeding, but the pulse is poor.

What happened? The pulse in the aorta above the graft is bounding, the pulse in the graft is greatly diminished, something is wrong. The anastamosis looks crimped, definitely not acceptable. There's no alternative, take down the proximal anastamosis and do it again. Give a bit more heparin, dissect a little higher; hate to do too much dissection as the patient is already heparinized. Ah, there's the problem, that thin back wall is cinched a bit, impeding proper flow. Let's do it again, hopefully, there won't be any problem. 3-0 prolene, let's go. There are no more pronouncements from across the table as we start back with the first new stitch at the 4:00 position. Ten minutes later we're done, or so we thought. The pulse is still poor; can't seem to get my act together. That thin back wall doesn't seem to be holding the stitches properly.

OK, a bit more dissection, now at the level of the renal arteries, the aorta is completely free and I think there is still a good cuff of aorta about 1.5 cm below the renal arteries. May need to divide the renal vein, but, no it is easily retracted out of the way. The aortic clamp is moved a bit higher, now situated so that it will be necessary to clamp right at the level of the renal arteries. The aorta is a bit ectatic (twisted, like the surgeon) and the clamp occludes the right renal artery, while the left remains open.

One more time, 3-0 prolene. Fifteen minutes later, after placing each bite of suture with as much careful precision as I can muster, I'm ready to tie the prolene and test the anastamosis, for the last time, I hope. With fingers and toes crossed the aortic clamp is released. The pulse is good and there is no leak, thank you Lord. Each leg is unclamped without difficulty, leaving only one more task.

The inferior mesenteric artery needs to be sewn back to the graft. The sigmoid colon definitely looks a bit blue (not depressed); blue as in ischemic. A cuff of aorta surrounding the IMA is cut and the newly placed aortic graft is partially clamped. The artery is quickly sewn to an opening in the graft and the clamp is removed. One little bit of bleeding is fixed with a single additional suture and there is a good pulse in the artery; normal pink color is restored to the colon and it looks like we've entered the homestretch.

2-0 Vicryl to close the posterior peritoneum, some minor bleeding from a small vessel in the fat, but otherwise no more surprises. The bowel all looks pink and is already peristalsing. The sigmoid colon no longer has that slightly bluish hue that was noted while the aorta was clamped; instead it is pink and healthy. #1 PDS for the fascia, irrigate the subcutaneous tissue, and leave the skin staples for my assistant.

As I walk away from the table the patients vital signs stare back at me, normal heart rate, blood pressure acceptable; all is well. I grab the chart and head to the ICU to dictate and write orders, and then to talk to his family. I wait in the ICU for the patient to arrive, five...ten minutes, plenty of time to get him packed up and wheeled from the first floor OR to the second floor ICU.

"Where's my patient?" I inquire of the OR front desk. "Still in Room 7? Is everything OK? I'll be down in a minute."

The patient is on his bed, but his blood pressure keeps fluctuating, falling as low as 65/40. Still, his heart rate is normal, his abdomen is not distended and I can feel his pulses OK. The anesthesiologist gives some medication in his IV, his blood pressure improves and he is quickly wheeled upstairs. *I don't think he's bleeding, Everything looked good when we finished* are my thoughts as I stand at the foot of his bed; the nurses are busy expertly plugging all the various monitors into their proper places. I nonchalantly feel his pulses while awaiting the report of his vital signs.

75/45 . . . 66 . . . O2 sat 99% . . . PA pressures 45/18 . . . CO 9L/min . . . SVR 450. Something is not right; those numbers suggest sepsis, unusual and unexpected in a fresh post-op aneurysm.

"We need an H & H right away and open up his fluids while we wait. Have some Dopamine and Levophed available."

These orders come from me as our very efficient ICU staff scurries about getting everything in order. Pressure is still low, still fluctuating between 60 and 80. What else to do? Back to surgery? Not yet, let's wait until we see the lab, give him some blood, fill up the tank.

The lab is OK, the H & H is higher than would be expected; bleeding seems less likely. There is a Swan Ganz catheter in place which may be useful in this situation. This type of intravenous catheter is threaded through a large central vein through the right side of the heart and into the pulmonary artery. Although the data obtained from this indwelling catheter is sometimes misleading it is useful to calculate cardiac output and it can provide a good indication of a patient's intravascular fluid status. What this all means is that it can help determine if a patient has too much fluid in their body or not enough.

In this case the numbers provided suggest that the patient is suffering from sepsis. This is a state that usually is a result of severe infection. The patient has a high cardiac output and low blood pressure. The systemic vascular resistance, which is a measure of the resistance faced by the heart as it pumps blood through the body's vessels is low. Such a state is very unusual in a freshly post op patient following Abdominal Aortic Aneurysm repair. Usually, it is the opposite state that exists.

Putting everything together, it seems to me that the patient probably received a bolus of bacteria after his colon was reperfused. During the surgery the aorta was clamped for about two hours, twice the normal time. The main vessel to the left side of the colon was clamped even longer as this was the vessel that had to be reimplanted after the graft was finally in place. It seems that this amount of time was enough for bacteria to cross the normal barriers that would have been disrupted as a result of the longer than normal clamp time. Although it is impossible to prove, this would explain everything.

The patient is finally becoming tenuously stable. His blood pressure is staying around 90 systolic and he is making some urine. His cardiac function is excellent. It's time to go to another surgery, an urgent case that has to be done today. Before I leave I explain everything to the patient's family. As soon as I arrive for the next surgery I call to the ICU; the patient is about the same.

After my next surgery, a repair of a pseudoaneurysm of a dialysis arterio-venous fistula, I head back to the ICU. The aneurysm patient is about the same, his blood pressure continues to fluctuate between 70 and 90 systolic. The pulmonary doctor is now there. A bit more blood transfused and he is now stabilizing at a BP of 90/40. It's now 7:30 pm and the patient has remained stable for thirty minutes. Talk to the family again and then home, at least for a short while.

An hour later I call for an update, BP is 90/50, heart rate is 70, he seems to be pretty stable. Great; it looks like he's turned the corner. Ten minutes later the strains of Pachobel's

Canon in D Major emanate from my phone; a message, call ICU stat.

The call is not good, the patient's suffered a cardiac arrest and they are doing CPR; some arrhythmias . . . cardiac origin . . . Dr. B is there . . . *OK, I'll be right in.*

So, I climb into the car and take the twenty minute drive back to the hospital, although this trip takes a bit less time. I arrive to find the patient with a BP of 90/45, HR 90 good oxygen saturation and Dr. B talking to his wife. A quick perusal of the patient reveals pupils equal in size, reactive to light, good femoral pulses, no abdominal distention. The last Hct is stable; unchanged from the one done a few hours before, in fact it is a little higher. Neither the exam nor the physiologic parameters suggest the patient is bleeding, rather sepsis is still suspected.

A long discussion with the patient's wife conveys two points: He's very sick and I don't think he needs to be returned to surgery. This last point goes against one of my unwritten rules: a hypotensive patient in the first few hours post surgery is assumed to be bleeding at a significant enough rate to warrant return to surgery unless proven otherwise. In this situation there are enough factors suggesting something other than bleeding; time to break the rules. Now just sit and wait and watch. He looks peaceful, almost serene, as the steady beeps of various monitors confirm his evolving stability.

So I take a little stroll, check on some other patients, and then wander back to the ICU. BP is a bit higher; amazingly, his urine output is pretty good, surprising in the face of two significant shocks to his kidneys; wait and watch a bit more.

Over the next few hours the patient becomes more stable, although requiring some support with pressors, continuous infusion of medication to maintain adequate blood pressure, ventilator support, and all the other usual therapeutic interventions typical to the septic ICU patient. The great, life-threatening danger seems to have passed; there is no more talk of returns to the OR or, as time passes, the possibility of not making it through. Dr. B and I discuss the patient each day as he continues to progress, goes to rehab for a few weeks and, finally, home almost back to normal.

The decision to not reoperate, in retrospect, was the correct one. If I had brought him back to surgery that first night would the outcome have been different? Would he have died? Or, would he have recovered more quickly? If I had returned him immediately to surgery, would he have suffered cardiac arrest or would he have arrested in the OR?

I'll never know the answers to these questions and it is one of the necessities of my profession that I not dwell on the consequences of each decision that is made. I often replay scenarios in my head and ask myself if I should have done something different. Hindsight is reported to be 20/20, but it is never quite that simple. Every time a surgeon picks up an instrument there are consequences. I always hope that what I do is for the patient's benefit. Even the simplest surgery creates changes in physiology that leaves the patient vulnerable to a number of potential complications. My job as surgeon is to perform the proper operation in a way that allows the patient to return to his normal state as quickly as possible.

When a patient "becomes sick" after an operation, all that can be done is to assess the situation on the merits of all available information, weigh all the different factors, and make a decision. At the same time, as situations evolve and factors change, decisions very often need to be altered. The knowledge and skills that a physician utilizes can only do so much. Our patients are who they are, with their own unique physiologic strengths and weaknesses, sometimes recovering because of what is done for them and sometimes in spite of it. And it is an unfortunate reality that far too often everything that a doctor can offer, all the medicine, surgery, and supportive measures in our vast arsenal is not enough and patients succumb.

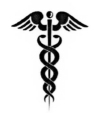

18. OR Ambience

Is this restaurant dead quiet or alive with noise? Perhaps it is simultaneously both until you open the door and enter.

—Erwin Schroedinger

Walk into an operating room and what will you see? If an operation is about to commence you will be greeted by bright lights, a variety of flashing lights, wires, tubes, hoses, stainless steel tables, and blue or green drapes adorning the star of the moment: the patient.

To the uninitiated visitor, operating room ambience can only be described in one way: sterile. Of course, it is absolutely essential that our operating theaters be perfectly sterile and most of the time this sterility is maintained. If the absolute cleanliness is breeched it is almost always the patient, by the nature of his or her disease that causes the break.

But, what of the ambience? The other day, while waiting to begin an operation, standing at the side of my already prepped and draped patient, I was struck by the sounds and sights that are common to almost every operating room;

sights and sounds that those of us who work in surgery take for granted and universally ignore.

The steady rhythm of the various monitors, EKG, and pulse oximeter, the intermittent whine of the inflating blood pressure cuff, the pumping of the ventilator are noises we expect and rarely notice. However, if the usual high pitch of the pulse oximeter falls to a lower note or the beeping of the EKG becomes very rapid or very slow I will usually glance up from my work and take a peek at the monitors and at the anesthesiologist. Is everything OK? Are these the sounds of a faulty lead? Or a real problem?

If the anesthesiologist is still nonchalantly thumbing his way through the *Wall Street Journal* or staring into his iPhone, I will assume that there isn't any problem, but I will usually ask, just to be on the safe side. Often a minor adjustment is all that is necessary to return the ambience to the usual expected state of monotony.

The sounds of anesthesia are usually regular and unchanging. The sounds of surgery, although rarely chaotic, are irregular and unpredictable. The mumblings of the surgeon as he asks for an instrument, the occasional slap of that instrument into the surgeon's palm, the beep and subsequent sizzle coming from the electrocautery are all noises that may be heard during even the most routine operation. Most of the time an observer would be treated to a workman-like and boring display with minimal excitement. Occasionally, there is some excitement; luckily it is an extremely occasional event. The occurrence of such rare events could possibly treat the spectator to the sight and sound of bleeding.

The sight of serious bleeding can be described as impressive, horrible, fearsome, and, most commonly, terrifying. An uncontrolled hole in a major artery will shoot blood up to the ceiling or across the room. The amount of pressure and force that our heart generates with each pump is enough to hit a spot many feet away. The soft whoosh of profound bleeding is the most dreadful sound that can be heard in the OR. At times like these a well placed finger usually provides at least a temporary fix; the proverbial finger in the dike.

Other sights common to surgery are tubes and wires running from here to there and back again. Tubing from the ventilator runs to a tube going through the patient's mouth and into the trachea. Bags of fluid hang on poles, relentlessly dripping into the patient's veins. Tubes run to various containers on the floor; one collecting urine, another to a canister collecting any bodily fluids caught by the suction device which keeps the operative field clear so the surgeon can actually see what he's doing and not be forced to operate by Braille.

The final sense that often is prominent in the OR is smell. The unique odors of surgery are often enough to scare even the most eager medical student into a life of radiology. The aforementioned electrocautery is used to stop bleeding from small blood vessels. It works by generating electrical current that heats the tissue and fills the blood vessel lumen with coagulated material, sealing the end of the vessel. The heat produces an odor of burning flesh as the tissue is coagulated. During laparoscopic surgery, where the cauterization is within the closed peritoneal cavity, the video image may become obscured by smoke that makes one think of London on a foggy night. At such a point the surgery is stopped and a valve opened to release the trapped smoke, sending up a plume that always reminds of the volcano at a Hibachi restaurant. Of course, it is customary to direct the smoke towards the head of the table, to the anesthesiologist, as they are used to breathing in noxious fumes.

Another notable fragrance, one similar to the odor of the cautery, is the distinct fragrance of heated bone when it is cut with a power saw. Now, I am no orthopedic surgeon, so there are few times when I am allowed access to their toys.

Most commonly this is as part of an amputation. In the early days of surgery amputation of limbs was, by far, the most common operation performed, utilizing primitive tools, the emphasis was on performing a speedy operation. However, modern times, with modern techniques and anesthesia allow for more leisurely procedures. Hand tools have given way to power and the unique smell of burning bone. I really don't know how to describe it, but it creates an ambience unique to the OR. Often, at least when I do amputations, there is an accompanying shower of fine droplets of blood.

Finally, the most memorable odor of the OR is the unforgettable aroma of a perforated colon, especially one that has been festering for several days. The mixture of bacteria, often combined with dead tissue that has been allowed to age for a few days, besides producing an extremely ill patient, creates a powerful smell that can permeate masks and gloves, often filling the entire OR with its unique pungency. At such times, OR personnel do their best to minimize this fetid fragrance so the operation can proceed without interruption. Oil of wintergreen or benzoin on the mask usually does the trick. Over the years many of my olfactory cells must have died off, because it is rare that I need any such assistance.

Although this olfactory delight is most common to a perforated colon, other conditions involving dead tissue and anaerobic or polymicrobial infection, such as perirectal abscesses and necrotizing perineal infection, can be just as potent.

Like a fine restaurant, the operating room has its own special ambience, one that attracts the finest people. In the course of attacking the most cruel diseases at their source these unique sights, sounds and smells pique our senses and keep us returning for more.

III. Postoperative

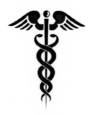

19. The Operation was a Success . . . but the Patient Died

'Tis not always in a physician's power to cure the sick; at times the disease is stronger than trained art.

—Ovid

The title above is a bit of a cliché, but, unfortunately it sometimes is true. Surgery has come a long way from the days of drilling holes in people's heads to let out evil spirits, and we have progressed well beyond the days of barbers as surgeons. The early days of surgery were marked by "the operation was a success, but the patient died" far too often.

Unfortunately, these modern days of surgery, with our knowledge of strict aseptic technique, minimally invasive surgery, and ambulatory procedures patients still can unexpectedly succumb after what seems to be a perfect operation. Why does this happen? Why should a patient who has just undergone an uneventful operation suddenly become very ill and die?

I wish I knew the answer; because if the answer was readily known such events could possibly be avoided. Patients die unexpectedly from undetected cardiac disease, blood clots that travel to the lungs, minor infections that turn out to be major, undetected bleeding, and a whole host of other conditions.

Sadly, I've seen unexpected post operative deaths far too often over the years. Perhaps it is the perfectionist in me, but I've always believed that if we surgeons do our job properly, sudden cardiac death, pulmonary emboli, and other complications would be banished to the back pages of textbooks, part of the chapter on history of surgery. But, we don't live in a perfect world, our patients are imperfect living organisms, and even the best surgeons are fallible human beings.

What can happen? Years ago, I performed an uneventful colon resection on Dan for a cancer in the cecum. The first morning after surgery I saw him on rounds, sitting up in a chair, minimal complaints of pain, no nausea, in short looking as well as could be expected one day post surgery. I left him and went to surgery without any concerns about his recovery; he was cruising through an uncomplicated post operative course. About an hour later I was writing orders for my just completed surgery when I heard an overhead page.

"Code Blue, Room 3023; Code Blue, Room 3023."

The room number seemed familiar and ten seconds later my phone rang and there was a message that Dan was coding; that is, he had suffered cardiopulmonary arrest. I raced up to the third floor and found the typical code scene, the ER physician running the show, the anesthesiologist taping in the just placed endotracheal tube, nurses calling out drugs and times, chest compressions in progress, and a distraught wife in the hallway wondering what was happening. I received a quick appraisal from the ER physician, took a glance at the monitor, and then sat down to talk to Dan's wife.

"It seems his heart has stopped," I explain. "They're doing all they can, but it doesn't look good." All she could do was silently cry and pray and hope as I left her to go check on Dan. It was obvious Dan wasn't going to make it and the code was halted. I had the difficult task of talking to Dan's wife and breaking the bad news.

"I'm sorry," are the word's I always use to start this task. "I'm sorry, but Dan didn't make it".

She started to cry and I put my hand on her shoulder; explained about his heart and it was unpredictable and was there anything else I could do, empty words that meant nothing and offered no solace. A nurse came to relieve me and I quickly left, feeling very inadequate and just a bit guilty. I didn't murder him, but if he hadn't undergone the operation he would probably still be alive, or, he may have had a heart attack anyway. But, there is no doubt that the surgery, even though indicated and necessary, hastened his demise.

A similar case, but luckily with a different outcome, was Glenn. Glenn was 78 years old and had a hernia. He was one of the few patients with an inguinal hernia that I repaired using laparoscopic technique. His pre-op EKG revealed a minor abnormality and he was referred to a cardiologist for cardiac evaluation and clearance for surgery. He had a normal stress test and was given the green light.

The surgery was for bilateral inguinal hernias and, being performed laparoscopically, required general anesthesia. The surgery lasted about ninety minutes, and when it was done and the patient was in recovery, his oxygen saturation was only 89% even with supplemental oxygen administration. A chest x-ray revealed pulmonary edema, which is fluid backing up into the lungs, often seen with heart failure. This was treated with Lasix, a diuretic which helps the body get rid of extra fluid. He improved, but developed persistent irregular heartbeats. His cardiologist was called and he underwent an emergency cardiac catheterization, which revealed that he had a 99% blockage of the left main coronary artery. Should that particular artery occlude completely, he likely would experience sudden death. The cardiac surgeon was called and Glenn had emergency heart bypass surgery and recovered uneventfully.

This case showed me that preoperative testing is never one hundred percent accurate and that surgery is a far greater stress test than the cardiologist's treadmill. Also, always suspect the worst possibility and be surprised and relieved when it doesn't develop.

A third example is Ethel. She was 86 years old and came to the emergency room with low blood pressure and abdominal distension. Her evaluation revealed a ruptured abdominal aortic aneurysm. Aneurysms are weakened areas on arteries that can burst like an overinflated balloon. Fifty percent of patients that suffer ruptured aortic aneurysms die suddenly and, if they make it to the hospital and to surgery, the chance of survival is about fifty percent, also. So Ethel had a ruptured AAA and my partner had been called. He does not do that type of surgery, so he called me.

Ethel was taken immediately to surgery and her aneurysm was repaired and she then went to the ICU. She had a prolonged stay, but gradually improved. She was reaching the point where we were considering moving her to the step-down unit when she pulled her feeding tube out of her nose, Normally, this is no great problem; merely replace it or give her a chance to eat on her own. In this case, however, she started bleeding from her nose. The blood pooled in the back of her throat, which she then aspirated (went into her lungs) and she died. All in a matter of minutes. Ethel had survived a very major surgery, multiple complications, and died anyway . . . of a nosebleed.

The operation was a success, but the patient died.

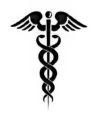

20. Sick Patients

Here's good advice for practice: Go into partnership with nature; she does more than half the work and asks none of the fee.

—Martin H. Fischer

At times during my ramblings I refer to patients becoming "sick." The non-medical person assumes that everyone that goes to the doctor, especially to a surgeon, is sick. Of course this is true, but the patients that I refer to as sick are those that share a common attribute: they have a life-threatening condition, known or unknown, that requires immediate and rapid attention and intervention.

When I first see a patient I begin my assessment as soon as I walk in the room. A patient sitting up smiling and laughing, bouncing around the bed is not "sick." A patient merely lying still, but otherwise comfortable is, also, probably not "sick", although may have a serious condition. However, the patient lying still, breathing rapidly, barely responding to questions or unresponsive, looking flushed or, even worse, ashen, may be "sick."

Such a patient requires immediate attention. If possible, a quick history from either the patient or a family member starts the physician down the proper path. Underlying illness, recent physical complaints, unusual behavior, any little abnormality helps steer in the right direction to establish a working diagnosis. In these situations, the physical exam can be most helpful. Rapid breathing and weak rapid pulse are hallmarks of the "sick" patient. Quick examination of the eyes, mouth, heart and lungs, abdomen, and extremities may help point to the etiology of the condition.

Scleral icterus, a hallmark of jaundice, may indicate liver failure; a tongue coated with the white spots of thrush suggest a compromised immune system possibly secondary to HIV disease or recent chemotherapy for cancer; distended neck veins along with crackles in the lungs suggest heart failure; a tender abdomen, visceral perforation or ischemia; mottled extremities, any or all of the above.

The causative factors vary from infection to trauma to heart failure, but in the severe state they lead to the same end: organ dysfunction and/or failure, the common final pathway for so many serious illnesses and the trademark feature of the "sick" patient.

In the distant past of medicine, say eighty years ago, such sick patients had one thing in common, they almost all died. In the days before antibiotics, dialysis, ventilators, inotropic pressor agents, total parenteral or even enteral nutrition, intravenous fluids, knowledge of fluid and electrolyte therapy and a host of other treatment modalities and interventions, there was very little that could be done for the patient with multi organ failure. Surgery was advanced enough in the 1930's that sometimes the offending organ could be repaired or removed and sometimes the patient would recover. Far more often, such patients would demonstrate initial improvement before ultimately succumbing to infection which led to massive organ failure.

Jump ahead to our modern times and there is a vast array of weapons to fight such diseases and support the sick patient through the worst phases of the disease process, buying time until the injured organ can recover and resume normal function.

The aforementioned ventilators, dialysis machines, powerful antibiotics, and patient specific fluid and electrolyte therapy join with high resolution CT scanners, MRI's, interventional radiology and minimally invasive surgery to treat the very sick patient in ways that were unimaginable fifty years ago.

Over the years I have seen more than my share of very sick patients. I started my post residency career as the Chief of the Trauma Service and Director of the Surgical Intensive Care Unit at Nassau County Medical Center on Long Island in New York. One of the memorable patients from those days was Juana, a survivor of a plane crash that left Avianca Flight 57 in a gully in the backyard of the parents of former tennis great, John McEnroe.

Juana was one of seventeen severely injured survivors of that plane crash that were brought to our hospital. I remember watching the local news in my home, which was across the street from the hospital; shortly after hearing the report of the crash, the phone rang and I was called to work.

The hospital was fully mobilized, even though it was nearly midnight. As the survivors rolled in they were quickly assigned to teams of surgeons and support staff. Juana had multiple orthopedic injuries, but no serious chest or abdominal injuries. Once she had been appropriately resuscitated she was taken to surgery by the Orthopedic team where she had a long operation fixing bilateral femur fractures, a fracture of the tibia and fibula and her left humerus. After surgery she was brought to the ICU where she was under the care of the Trauma Service.

Needless to say, she had a stormy ICU stay, suffering from respiratory failure, sepsis secondary to Candida (yeast), and renal failure. She was so "sick" that the Chief Resident on my service notified the local organ procurement organization that her demise was imminent and that she could be a potential donor, although her systemic disease was so bad there wouldn't be much to salvage. Personally, I thought the Chief Resident was a bit premature in his assessment and, sure enough, Juana proved him wrong.

She suffered through a difficult course of Amphotericin B, a toxic antifungal medication, severe Adult Respiratory Distress Syndrome, renal failure, but never needed dialysis and gradually recovered, completely; a sick patient who left the hospital "well."

Over the years supportive therapy for such patients has improved. One condition that can be very unforgiving, no matter how good the treatment, is pancreatitis or inflammation of the pancreas. The pancreas is a multifunctional organ that sits behind the stomach, sort of spongy to feel. It makes a number of important hormones, insulin being the most well known, as well as producing the enzymes that help digest our food. When someone develops pancreatitis their symptoms can range from mild pain and nausea to overwhelming, life-threatening sepsis.

Pancreatitis allows the digestive enzymes that are normally secreted into the duodenum, the first part of the small intestine, to leak out of the pancreas into the surrounding tissue. The body starts to digest itself. This process often leads to the fat surrounding the pancreas being digested into a thick paste of soap. Very often pancreatitis is associated with high levels of triglycerides in the blood. The blood of these patients literally looks like pink cream. It is easy to imagine the derangement our circulatory system suffers under these conditions. The resulting organ dysfunction is devastating.

Lungs, kidneys, brain, muscle, everything goes haywire. The causes of pancreatitis are numerous, but alcohol ingestion, gallstones, and severe hyperlipidemia (elevated levels of fat in the blood) are the most common etiologies.

For example, the case of Johnny stands out. Johnny was a young, robust man, 32 years old, alcoholic, who was admitted with severe pancreatitis. From the start of his illness, he had most of the signs that suggested that he was in for a stormy course. In addition, he started to go through alcohol withdrawal just as the pancreatitis was revving up. As all these processes started to wreak havoc on his body, his mind started to play games. He started to see large rats running along the walls of the ICU. When the nurses called me to see him, we tried to assure him that he was safe, but the rats won out and he jumped out of bed and ran from the ICU, stark naked, with his urinary catheter dragging between his legs. He stopped in a corner of one of the medical floors armed with a solid metal IV pole.

Security was called to help corral our wayward patient, but as they arrived Johnny started swinging his weapon back and forth and the guards prudently took a step back. The standoff continued for about twenty minutes until one of the older (and wiser) nurses appeared. She gently approached Johnny, gown in hand, and whispered in his ear, "John, you're naked and there are a lot of women around." He gave a sheepish grin and tried to cover himself.

She gave him the gown and led him back to the ICU.

Unfortunately, Johnny only got sicker. Twelve hours later he needed ventilator support, he developed renal failure and became comatose and ultimately died, a victim of his own excesses.

Patients like Juana and Johnny are encountered every day. They populate ICU's from Honolulu to Boston. The doctors that care for them do all they can, supporting each system to the maximum while waiting for the damaged body to start to heal itself. All that is done, every medication that is given, every tube that is placed, every X-ray or CT scan may not be enough. Like Johnny, sick patients die.

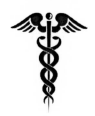

21. Don't Think

Constant attention by a good nurse may be just as important as a major operation by a surgeon.
—Dag Hammarskjold

I read a missive from hospital administration recently posted on the wall in the physicians work area at one of the hospitals. The message read something along these lines:

"Per JCAHO regulations, physicians should refrain from writing orders allowing for a range of medication to be administered. Specifically, pain medication orders should not say:

Dilaudid 1-2 mg IV Q3h prn pain

Instead such orders should be written:

Dilaudid 1 mg IV Q3h prn moderate pain
Dilaudid 2 mg IV q3h prn severe pain

Orders written in the former manner, allowing for a range of dosage, allow the nurse administering the medication to make independent judgment decisions. Such decision-making is not permitted under the nursing licensure."

My reaction to this directive was that the lunatics are in charge of the asylum and everyone should run for cover. Nurses are to become robots, methodically passing out meds and dutifully charting when the patient last belched, while ignoring their patient's overall wellbeing. I asked several of the nurses in various hospitals their opinion of this rule. I pointed out that, to me, there wasn't any difference between the two orders. What they said was a bit disconcerting. The nurse is supposed to ask the patient about the severity of their pain and then medicate accordingly. So, if the patient responds that he is feeling severe pain he is given the higher dose, no questions asked.

Now, I've been in practice for over twenty years and I can tell you that pain; its intensity, quality, severity, and every other aspect is the most subjective of clinical symptoms. I've had patients, who have undergone a very minor procedure, tell me the pain is the most excruciating they've ever felt, while others, who have just undergone a major abdominal surgery with a stem to stern incision, report only mild discomfort.

There are patients who appear nearly comatose after surgery, barely arousable, but will state that their pain is severe and will request their medication every three hours on the dot. In this situation, what is the nurse to do? Blindly administer the higher dose prescribed for severe pain or actually think that the patient's pain may not be as severe as reported and give the lower dose, and/or call the doctor to have the medication adjusted.

No matter what, a good nurse has to use her best judgment to care for her patient in the most compassionate, but also clinically appropriate, manner possible. Patients, who are mostly human, have widely varying ideas of what the hospital experience should be, particularly when it comes to pain. For some, pain relief means completely numb from head to toe; for others it means just enough medication to have the edge taken off. Most are somewhere in the middle. The nurse serves as the doctor's eyes, learns to make a proper judgment and provides a continuous image that complements the snapshot the doctor receives on daily rounds.

The idea that nurses not be allowed to think echoes the words of one of my medical school instructors, Dr. John Adams (see the chapter "Tension"). In the early 1980's I was at the University of Rochester Medical School in upstate New York. Dr. Adams was the classic curmudgeonly surgeon. Loud, intolerant of ignorance or incompetence by subordinates, he often chastised the residents on his service for writing orders with a dosage range in the way that is now prohibited. He must be working for the JCAHO, because his exact words were:

"Don't write Demerol 50-75 mg IM q3h. That allows the nurse to think; we don't want the nurses to think. Their job is to do what they are told to do."

Who would have thought chauvinistic Dr. Adams was such a visionary?

Actually, I don't think that he had such a low opinion of nurses; rather, I believe, he was trying to drive home a message to the residents and students: Orders should be clear and specific. Such clarity allows the nurse to perform her task efficiently and provide the patient with the best care possible. Doctors and nurses are a team, working together to help an individual who is sick or injured recover and return to a normal life.

Years ago I read a study on factors affecting outcomes on critically ill patients. I don't remember which journal it was in, but the study looked at ICU patients and a number of variables that could have an effect on the patient's recovery. The only variable that made any difference was the quality of nursing care.

This makes perfect sense to me. The critically ill patient requires continuous monitoring. Most of the time it is the nurse that is at the bedside checking vital signs, urine output, oxygenation, and every other parameter that may be indicative of the patients well-being. The best ICU nurses will pick up on subtle changes that could be harbingers of impending deterioration in the patient's clinical condition. If such nurses are shackled by the "don't think and don't make judgment" rules, these critically ill patients will suffer.

Besides acting as physicians' eyes, nurses also provide a level of protection for the patient. If an order is written or a medication prescribed that seems to be in error, the nurse is there to question it. Despite what some doctors may believe, we physicians are not perfect and sometimes errors are made. A vigilant nurse often picks up on this, questioning the order and calling the doctor for a "clarification" (correction). Sometimes it is an omission that needs to be brought to the doctor's attention. In all situations the nurse is the patient's advocate, doing his or her best to smooth the often bumpy road to recovery.

Doctors, by necessity, approach patient care from a very different angle than nurses. Medical School and residency teach us the underlying pathophysiology and the clinical manifestations of various diseases and medical conditions. We take this information and establish a diagnosis and institute a therapeutic plan. Our primary purpose is to see that the disease process is properly treated and see the patient to a complete recovery, or at least keep chronic diseases under control.

Nurses share in this goal, but along the way they are often called upon to provide comfort, counseling and to allay fears. The nature of their profession allows nurses to do this in a way doctors cannot. The best nurses always seem to find the time to sit with their patients, provide reassurance and still manage to do all the ridiculous charting and filling out of seemingly endless forms that generate reams of paper that no one ever looks at.

In the middle of these essential activities, nurses often have their carefully planned schedules disturbed by a million other tasks, usually accommodating the interruptions with a smile and a shrug of the shoulders. I know that when I have asked nurses to help with a bedside procedure, they are only eager to help and always insist on finishing up all the cleaning and reordering of the patient room when I am finished. I sometimes wonder if it is eagerness to do all they can to help or if they really want to be sure that the patient's room is properly returned to an orderly state.

Nurses are truly amazing in their ability to calm anxiety, inform ignorance, allay fear, provide comfort, stroke egos (especially OR nurses), see us all at our worst moments, and invade our most intimate places, and do it all with a smile and a wink that says, "I know you don't feel well now, but just give us a little time and you'll back home with your loved ones before you know it."

I may be a bit biased towards nurses. After all, I married one; Laura, my wonderful, beautiful, intelligent wife of twenty five years, the cutest little nurse I had ever seen, always took the time to talk to her patients, share their feelings, and make sure that all their treatment was delivered in the best, most professional manner. When we first met I think I used to exasperate her by my asking for patients' vital signs and her appraisal of their condition. But, we shared our concern for the patients' well being and have continued to share for twenty five years.

Nurses and doctors, along with respiratory therapists, physical therapists, occupational therapists, speech pathologists, patient care aids, and all the other allied health personnel, share a common goal; that is to treat the sick and injured and allow them to return to happy, healthy, productive lives. The doctor provides the diagnosis and overall therapeutic plan, institutes the plan's delivery, and makes alterations and interventions when necessary. The nurse provides the monitoring, the immediate delivery of therapy, nurturing, comforting and compassion on a continuous basis. If our nurses are not allowed to "think" our patients will end up suffering, with longer stays in the hospital and some, I am sure, will never leave the hospital.

It is something for all of us to think about.

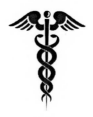

22. Memorable

A memory is what is left when something happens and does not completely unhappen.

—Edward de Bono

After so many years in the trenches of surgery there are some cases that stick in my head, memorable for one reason or another. Patients with unusual presentations, unexpected outcomes (good and bad), or just out of the ordinary. Many of these have already been discussed elsewhere in these pages, but here are a few more.

William was a patient admitted with a ruptured abdominal aortic aneurysm. He was in his fifties, a heavy smoker, and drove a truck for a living. I was the sixth surgeon down the list to be called; none of the first five were available. I had been on my way to do another surgery when the call came, so I turned around and headed back to the previous hospital. He was a typical patient that had survived the initial rupture to make it to the hospital. His blood pressure varied between 70/0 and 90/50. After quickly assessing the situation I called up to the OR and asked, I guess a bit nonchalantly, if they were busy. One of the tech's answered the phone, thinking I wanted to schedule an appendectomy or some other routine add-on.

I said, in a rather flat voice, "Well, I've got this patient with a ruptured aortic aneurysm I need to do right away."

Silence was the initial reply and then she exclaimed, "You're joking, right?"

"No," I replied, "it's definitely ruptured and I need to go right away."

"Oh, shit, I'll call you right back."

Well, we got him to surgery in short order and he had the smoothest ruptured aneurysm repair I had ever done, less than two hours, start to finish. Two days after surgery he looked like nothing had happened, off the ventilator, breathing on his own, kidneys working normally. I thought that he'd be home in less than a week. Of course, it didn't go that way. His heavy smoking history caught up with him and he developed pulmonary problems which progressed to full blown Adult Respiratory Distress Syndrome. He was reintubated and went back on the ventilator, developed renal failure, sepsis secondary to Candida (yeast), and looked to be at death's door. He became so ill, with almost every organ system failing, that his wife decided to withdraw support, which would have meant to let him die. She actually signed the papers and plans were made to take him off the ventilator. Fortunately, six hours later, she changed her mind. Supportive care was maintained and over the next three weeks he improved. His sepsis resolved with therapy, his renal function recovered, and he was eventually able to breathe on his own. About four weeks after his initial surgery, he walked out of the hospital. Only the persistence of William's wife allowed him to survive as he surely would have succumbed if supportive measures were withdrawn.

A quite different story was Doug. Poor Doug was out driving his truck one evening, drinking, and came to a fork in the road. One way lead to his home and his wife, while the other lead to his girlfriend's apartment. Apparently, he couldn't decide which one he wanted to see that night and so he didn't take either fork and instead went straight, right into a tree. When he arrived in the ER our evaluation revealed some broken ribs, a fractured pelvis, and a closed head injury. He was minimally responsive and required endotracheal intubation and ventilator support. The only surgery he needed was a tracheostomy about ten days into his ICU stay. He gradually improved, woke up, and his consciousness became nearly normal.

After about four weeks, he seemed well enough to be transferred out of the ICU. He was breathing on his own, although he still had his tracheostomy tube in place, which meant that he was breathing through a tube that went through a hole in his neck directly into his windpipe. The tube had a balloon around it that sealed his airway away from his mouth and nose. After he'd been out of the ICU for about twelve hours I heard a "code blue" called on the surgical floor and then the call came to me. Doug had arrested, his tracheostomy tube had become plugged and he had suffocated. Despite all efforts, he did not survive.

This case sticks in my mind for several reasons, mostly because Doug's transfer with his tracheostomy tube in place and the balloon cuff inflated was a great error in judgment. While in the ICU, Doug was monitored 100% of the time. If any problem arose, a nurse was right there to address it. On the floor, however, he was on his own, more or less. With the tracheostomy tube in place and the balloon cuff inflated, he couldn't speak and even though he was recovering from his head injury he still was not adept enough to push the call bell for the nurse. When his tube became plugged there were no monitors to alert the nurse and he was unable to call for help; he couldn't yell out and he was unable to even push the button. His was a death that shouldn't have happened. If he had been transferred with just the balloon cuff deflated, he probably would have been fine, as he would have been able to breath around the plugged up tracheostomy tube. Ever since this avoidable death, I have never sent a patient to an unmonitored bed with a tracheostomy balloon inflated.

Roxanne came to me complaining of a lump in her breast. She had noticed it for several months and it had increased slightly in size. Her Primary Care Physician had seen her and ordered a mammogram which was reported as normal. A few months passed, the mass persisted, and she was referred to me. Roxanne was in her mid forties, obese, but otherwise healthy. When I examined her there was a definite mass in the upper inner part of her left breast, large enough for me to do a biopsy right then and there. The needle biopsy was positive for cancer and she elected to undergo mastectomy with immediate reconstruction. She saw the Plastic Surgeon and the combined procedure was scheduled for the following week.

The surgery went smoothly, everything healed adequately, and she recovered uneventfully. She returned eight months later with a new lump in her reconstructed breast. Biopsy was done and it showed recurrent cancer. The options were more limited now. She underwent a mastectomy of the reconstructed breast, followed by radiation therapy and chemotherapy. After everything had healed and she finished her other therapy, she disappeared from my practice.

Eight years later I saw her name on my schedule, coming to see me for gallbladder disease. I wasn't sure it was the same Roxanne, but when she walked through the door

I recognized her immediately. She underwent an uneventful cholecystectomy and then disappeared again. Five years later she reappeared with a different, minor problem.

Roxanne is memorable because she was an unexpected survivor. Young women with aggressive breast cancer usually succumb to their disease at an early age. It is always gratifying to me when a patient who has cancer (or any such life-threatening disease), and has undergone extensive surgery and then disappears into the hands of the Radiation or Medical Oncologist for therapy, shows up years later, free of disease. It tells me that, sometimes everything we do is worth it. Extensive disfiguring surgery, followed by the poison of chemotherapy, really has some benefit. The Medical Oncologist frequently gets to see the fruits of his labor (also the failures), but this is not so true for the surgeon. The treatment very often starts with a surgeon's scalpel, but afterward the patient is lost to us. A patient such as Roxanne, surviving despite the odds, always brings a smile to my face.

Chad and Bill are two patients I always think of together. They both had extensive surgery for cancer, developed complications, but survived. Chad had undergone a "Whipple" procedure for cancer of the pancreas; the surgery actually performed by one of my partners with my assistance. Two days after the surgery my partner left for a three-week vacation and I assumed Chad's care. He developed complications which required a return to surgery and required several drainage procedures.

Bill had a complex surgery performed by one of the urologists, for bladder cancer. About a week into the post operative period he was found to have GI contents (feces) draining through his incision, always a cause for some alarm. I was consulted and he was returned to the Operating Room and had a portion of his small intestine removed. This surgery was performed by me and his care then became my responsibility.

Bill was in ICU Bed 2 and Chad was in Bed 11. Over the next three months I started each day going from Bed 2 to Bed 11 as they gradually recovered. Chad developed leakage of bile which gradually healed. Bill had respiratory failure complicated by his pre-existing lung disease. Chad recovered first and left the hospital after three and a half months. Bill finally was able to get out of the hospital after five months.

These two patients are memorable for several reasons. They were in the hospital at the same time and stayed in the ICU for a long time. Both had cancer and, unfortunately, both had recurrence of their cancer at about the same time. Bill returned only six weeks after his discharge with a large mass in his right lung, which was malignant and had caused a lung abscess. He died about one month later. Chad fared a little better. His pancreatic cancer recurred three months after he was discharged, did not respond to any treatment, and he died two months later.

But they are memorable to me for one other reason. They are the first patients I ever asked about their recollection of the prolonged ICU stay each had experienced. They answered in almost identical manner. What they remembered:

"The entire stay is a fog. It's like several months of my life have been lost, simply vanished from consciousness. I don't remember any visits, any pain, or anything."

I think our bodies, or perhaps something higher, provide remarkable defense mechanisms. An experience that has to be incredibly painful is completely wiped away, saving the patient, victim, or whoever the pain of reliving it over and over. Psychiatrists would say that it is submerged in the subconscious and will emerge in some manifestation years later. Bill and Chad never had the opportunity. Still, they did recover enough to have some meaningful time out of the hospital before succumbing to their disease.

And then there's Cliff. Over the years I have taken care of a number of patients that have jumped from high places and failed to fly; unable to defy the law of gravity, they plummet to the ground until their sudden deceleration and collision with the Earth inflicts injury.

Cliff stands out among all the jumpers. He made his first appearance in the ER after he slashed his wrists, an obvious suicide gesture. A less than stellar ER clerk or triage nurse instructed him to wait in the lobby. Apparently perturbed by the lack of attention, he left the ER and decided to perform a more extravagant act to get the attention he deserved. He managed to jump from an eleventh-story window and smash through a car windshield.

He was returned to our ER and I started my resuscitation and survey of the damage. My first thoughts were, "What will we operate on first?" He did have severe injuries. He was immediately intubated to secure an airway and he required chest tubes as treatment for bilateral hemopneumothoraces (collapsed lungs with bleeding into the space around the lung). He had fractured eleven vertebrae, but he was neurologically intact. He had a fractured pelvis which was deemed stable by the orthopedic service and his peritoneal lavage was negative for any bleeding into his abdomen.

Despite his best efforts, Cliff, at least initially, didn't need any surgery. He was admitted to the ICU and gradually recovered from his injuries. He eventually did need an operation. He developed acute cholecystitis and underwent a cholecystectomy about three weeks into his hospital stay. When I left that particular service he was up walking with physical therapy and he eventually left the hospital, walking and talking, completely normal.

Finally, there is a patient who is memorable for many reasons. Rico came to my office with a diagnosis of hemorrhoids, which is swelling of tissue around the anus. Examination quickly revealed that his condition was far more serious than uncomplicated hemorrhoids. He had a mass protruding through his anus that was hard and bled at the slightest touch. A biopsy was done and it revealed he had adenocarcinoma of the rectum, that is, rectal cancer.

He received initial treatment with a single dose of radiation therapy, the protocols for treatment at the time were not as clearly defined as they are today, followed by surgery, an abdominoperineal resection. This is an extensive operation that removes the rectum and anus, and leaves the patient with a permanent colostomy. His tumor was very advanced and the surgery required removing tissue from around the rectum which included stripping the capsule from the prostate gland which is adjacent to the rectum. This maneuver led to uncontrollable bleeding and my only option was to pack his pelvis, which put pressure against the bleeding gland and stopped the bleeding. At this point the plan was to leave the packing in place for 48 hours, allow the offending organ to stop bleeding as the oozing vessels clot, and then return to the OR, remove the packs, and hope that all had gone as planned. It turned out that this worked as expected and he left the hospital about a week later.

However, two weeks later he came to the office complaining of abdominal pain, nausea, and vomiting. He went back into the hospital and x-rays revealed small bowel obstruction, a blockage in the small intestine. A tube was passed through his nose into his stomach to "decompress" his blocked intestines and then we waited. Most patients that develop a small bowel obstruction in the first few weeks after surgery will respond to such therapy, the blockage will resolve without surgery and they recover uneventfully. But, Rico just wasn't like other patients. After several days it was apparent that he wasn't going to open up and he was returned to surgery again. The obstruction was caused by his small intestine slipping down into his pelvis, into the space that was previously occupied by his rectum. The trapped bowel was released and I did what I could to prevent a recurrence.

Fortunately, he didn't have any more problems and recovered uneventfully. Besides this complicated course, I remember Rico because I see him almost every day. He works as a custodian at several of the hospitals where I practice. Every time he sees me he waves, clasps his hands together and says, reciting some of the few English words that he knows, "God bless you, Doctor, bless you." He is cured of his cancer, I presume. His surgery was more than ten years ago. I sometimes wonder why God chose this man to be a survivor. By all indicators, his cancer should have recurred, the tumor was huge and was invading outside the rectum. Although I did a very generous resection, similar cases usually recurred. Whatever the reasons, he is a daily reminder of the good that doctors can do, that a situation that seems to be hopeless doesn't have to be, and that God works in His own mysterious ways.

I'm not sure why some cases are memorable and some are forgotten. Often the memorable case involves an error by someone, usually me, but it could be anyone or anything that leaves me with the feeling that this particular patient should have been treated differently or should have had a different outcome. Or, as my old Chief of Surgery, Dr. Dibenedetto, often responded when asked how he could remember some minute detail, "Some things are just memorable, you just don't forget, you know?" How right he was.

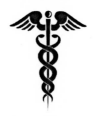

23. *Heard In and Around the OR*

Muffled lives explode in understatements.

—Paul Gray

In Pre-op:

The pre-op nurse will ask, "What surgery are you having today?"

"Repair of my hi-anal hernia." (Hiatal Hernia.)

"Doctor is going to remove the fireballs from my eucharist." (Fibroids of the Uterus.)

"Fix my piles." (Hemorrhoids.)

"Suck out my gallbag." (Laparoscopic Cholecystectomy.)

"Fix my erotic aneurysm." (Aortic Aneurysm.)

When asked, "What's your surgeon's name?"

"I don't know, he's the one with red hair and glasses."

Before starting surgery:

When a general surgeon says, "This will only take thirty minutes," it means, "It will take me thirty minutes assuming this tumor is in the sigmoid colon where the GI doc said it's supposed to be. However, it could be in the stomach instead of the colon, so call Dr. Smith, who's following my case, and tell him he'll have plenty of time for lunch."

When an Orthopedic surgeon says, "This will only take thirty minutes," it means, "We'll fix this and then get an x-ray and then do it again until I figure out which bone is connected to what; it will be at least three hours."

When a plastic surgeon says, "This will only take thirty minutes," it means, "It will take me thirty minutes to set up my camera. The surgery will probably four or five hours."

Things heard during surgery and what they really mean.

Anesthesiologist to surgeon: "Is everything OK down there?"

Translation: "The EKG is flat, there's no blood pressure, and you'd better start CPR."

Surgeon to anesthesiologist: "We're having a little blood loss."

Translation: "I just cut the vena cava and you'd better call the blood bank, get the cell saver and a priest."

Surgeon to no one in particular: "That's not supposed to be there."

Translation: "Call my lawyer, malpractice carrier and my mother, I just cut the Common Bile Duct."

Surgeon to anesthesiologist: "He's waking up."

Translation: "Put down the *Wall Street Journal* and turn up the gas before the patient walks off the table."

Surgeon to OR crew: "This is a new procedure; it may take a bit longer than usual."

Translation: "I've only seen this done once before and I was hung over at the time."

Surgeon to assistant: "This is a particularly difficult case."

Translation: I haven't the foggiest notion of how to proceed. Take over, I'm going to the bathroom."

Circulating nurse to surgeon: "We're out."

Translation: "You don't need that, you old fool, and even if you do, I'm not walking all the way to Room 12 to get it."

Surgeon to anesthesiologist: "Put another quarter in your machine."

Translation: "I've got at least another hour to work and the patient is awake enough to assist me."

Anesthesiologist to surgeon: "This patient's very high risk, but I think we can manage."

Translation: "I've got vacation coming up and business has been slow."

Soft "whoosh" . . . (Silence).

Translation: I've just cut the (choose one or all) aorta, inferior vena cava, and portal vein." The "whoosh" is the sound of bleeding; the silence is the sense of doom. It is permissible to replace the silence with "Oh Shit!" Or any other similar epithet.

Such utterances are, fortunately, extremely rare. When something unexpected happens the greatest effort is made to maintain a calm, workmanlike atmosphere which explains the tendency to seemingly understate the gravity of the situation. As long as channels of communication are maintained between the members of the OR crew, the patient will receive the utmost attention.

Feel free to add to the list.

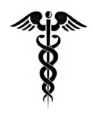

24. The End of Life

God pours life into death and death into life without a drop being spilled.

—Author Unknown

It is one of the undeniable facts of life that from the moment of our birth we are destined to die. As a doctor I have, unfortunately, been intimately involved with dozens of deaths over the years. The manner that any individual passes from our world is the product of multiple factors.

Over the years I have noticed that the dying process comes in many forms; sometimes sudden and, more often, gradual. Most deaths that I witness seem to come with the individual failing in parts, a little bit at a time. I frequently am called to attend to a patient with a portion of their body suffering a specific manifestation of a disease process. Other specialists also may be called, depending on the body part or system that is affected.

If the brain dies first, that is, a patient suffers a stroke, the Neurologist or Neurosurgeon is called. A dying leg is addressed by the vascular surgeon; the heart, a Cardiologist;

intra-abdominal organ, General Surgeon, and so on. We often die a piece at a time which may allow for a temporary reversal of the process. It is the physician's task to restore these individual parts to proper working order and, as a result, restore the entire apparatus.

The causes of these disruptions of organs and organ systems are as numerous as the myriad of diseases that exist. Occlusions of blood vessels that feed vital organs lead to heart attacks, strokes, or gangrene of various organs with resultant sudden death, disability, or, hopefully, recovery. Traumatic injury, tumors, chemical intoxication, or infections are other causative factors that lead to organ dysfunction or demise.

Doctors that are called upon to intervene employ a vast armamentarium to stem and reverse the progression of such disease, most often with great success and the specter of death is left outside, looking in, an unwelcome visitor forced to return another day.

But, there are times when we fail; times when we know that the end is inevitable. It is at these times a doctor's skill and compassion are most challenged. After all, we are taught that death is the enemy. Our job is to cure our patients, to return them to normal, happy, productive lives, and anything short of this is failure, forces us to confront our own humanity with all its limitations.

Although I am frequently amazed at the resiliency of the human body I am just as often reminded of its fragility. When all efforts have been exhausted and there is only one inevitable outcome, physicians are called upon to ease the fears and suffering of our patients and their families and, we hope, help bring peace to their final days or moments.

There are two specific patients I cared for in the past that illuminate this final point with great clarity. The first was Dorothy, a woman of eighty, mother of seven and a deeply religious Christian. I first encountered her when she was admitted to the hospital with gallbladder disease. At that time she had an uneventful surgery and went home in short order. Several months later she returned much sicker with a blockage in her small intestine. All efforts to treat her without surgery were unsuccessful and she underwent another operation.

At surgery she was found to have widespread cancer caused by a tumor that originated in her small intestine, an unusual type of cancer; in this case incurable. I performed a palliative procedure, relieving the intestinal obstruction and informed her and her family that it was likely the disease would progress, she possibly would suffer future obstructions and that she would likely die within a period of months. Chemotherapy was offered which would possibly slow the progression of disease, but with very little hope for cure. This was politely declined and she left the hospital under the care of hospice.

Almost exactly two years later she was readmitted with progressive weakness, but little pain and no evidence of recurrent intestinal obstruction. It was apparent that she had reached her final days. Her seven sons and daughters were notified, and a few days later she succumbed, peacefully, all of her family at her bedside.

In contrast to this anecdote, there is another, much shorter one, to recount. As chief resident in surgery at Nassau County Medical Center on Long Island I was responsible for pretty much any patient that came into the hospital that needed surgery. In particular, Nassau County was the major trauma center for the area.

On this particular day the familiar, "Trauma team to the trauma room; Trauma team to the trauma room," was heard overhead. The team on call, with me in charge, stood by waiting for the arrival of a serious boating accident. After about 10 minutes, Michael arrived, typically agitated, but awake and alert. He was able to talk but gave us few details of the accident other than the boat he was in had exploded and he had been thrown a great distance into the water. His vital signs were fairly normal, in fact his blood pressure was very high, 170/100. The typical resuscitative measures began and a quick physical survey followed, and I noted that, although the pulses at his wrists and neck were normal, I could not feel any femoral pulses. Michael complained about pain in his chest and a rapidly performed chest x-ray confirmed my suspicions. I called the operating room and my Thoracic Surgery attending.

The chest x-ray revealed that the left chest was whited out, which suggested massive bleeding into the left chest and all but confirming my provisional diagnosis of a thoracic aorta injury. Michael remained very agitated as he was wheeled up to surgery. As I spoke to the attending, his only comment was, "Oh shit, I'm on my way."

As we wheeled into the OR, Michael's blood pressure had fallen to 70/0, but he was still awake and very agitated, as if he knew that something was terribly wrong and his end was imminent. He suffered cardiac arrest as he was placed on the operating room table, at which point I took a scalpel, opened up his chest and was greeted by almost his entire blood volume spilling out onto me, drenching me from chest to feet. I vainly clamped his ascending aorta while trying to find the tear, but all for naught. Despite expeditious treatment, Michael succumbed to a lethal injury.

After all this, it was my duty to inform his waiting family, a mother and sister who had been with him as he was wheeled up to surgery, awake and talking. They were now forced to face the reality of his untimely and unexpected death. The sad, anguished reply was much crying and screaming; a young person suddenly taken away to a premature fate is never calmly received.

These two scenarios present the extremes of the spectrum. One peaceful and calm, the other violent and disturbing. Doctors deal with both extremes and all the intermediate possibilities at one time or another. Some do it better than others. As a general surgeon I frequently face diseases that progress rapidly and I'm often the first to inform patients and their families that they have cancer or some other dreaded condition. Other specialists deal with other chronic diseases, but everyone ultimately ends the same. I truly believe, however, that how one dies is far more important than why one dies. Doctors do all they can to affect the why, but it is just as important to pay attention to the how.

We have made great strides in this area. We have been taught the five stages of dying, hospices are available to keep the terminal patient comfortable and even the health care reform act addresses this issue. In the end, such decisions are best left to the patient and families, with doctors, nurses and other medical personnel serving an important advisory role. In particular, the attending physician should inform the patient and family on diagnosis, prognosis, expected clinical scenarios and treatment options. Armed with such information the patient or family, if the patient is incapacitated, can make an educated decision.

I'm not sure that there is a point to these ramblings about the end of life. Death is just another reality of life, one we all have to face sooner or later. Our beliefs and life circumstances dictate how we respond. It can be viewed as a release from pain, the beginning of a new journey, an endless sleep or a violent end; one to be avoided at all cost or a time to receive the reward promised in so many religious scriptures.

We can never know for sure what awaits us, but I believe that Blaise Pascal had it right. We can't be sure what awaits us, but we should hope for the best; however, a little insurance never hurts.

*In brief, Pascal's wager stated that there are two possibilities and two choices. The possibilities are that God exists or that God does not exist. The choices are to believe in God (and Jesus) or to not believe in God. If God does not exist, then at death the individual is dead, gone, finished whether he believed in God or not.

If God does exist, then at the time of death the believer receives salvation while the unbeliever suffers eternal damnation. Pascal believed that given the options it made the most sense to believe in God and accept His Son as Savior.

IV. THE LIGHTER SIDE

Surgical training is accomplished through residency programs. Such training was first instituted by William Halsted, the first Chief of Surgery at Johns Hopkins Hospital, and the trainees were truly residents. They literally lived in the hospital and were available at any hour to attend to patient needs. Over the years surgical residencies have seen the hours spent caring for patients and time in the OR diminish. In recent years the number of residents applying for full training in general surgery has decreased and new residency rules have diluted the training experience.

The next two chapters address this growing problem in surgery.

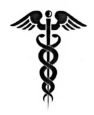

25. *Surrogate Surgery*

Standardization of our educational systems is apt to stamp out individualism and defeat the very ends of education by leveling the product down rather than up.
—Harvey Cushing quote

It was announced today that a pilot program is commencing in Baltimore under provisions covered on page 2438 of the new Health Care Reform Act. It is anticipated that there will be considerable shortage of general surgeons in the years to come. Incomplete filling of residency rosters coupled with the aging population will lead to a deficit of over 10,000 general surgeons over the next 20 years.

This deficit is expected to hit hardest in rural areas, but many urban areas are already experiencing many weeks without adequate emergency and, at times, even elective coverage for many specialties, but particularly in the very important area of general surgery.

This section of the Health Care Act provides for coverage by health care providers that act as surrogates for the traditional physician or surgeon. Nurse practitioners, physician assistants, nurse midwives, and similar health care providers all are anticipated to play vital roles insuring that quality healthcare is delivered to many underserved areas.

The new program, called the Simian Surrogate Program or SSP, is undertaking the task of training apes to perform many of the operations now performed by general surgeons. Specifically, chimpanzees and orangutans are currently undergoing intense education in surgical technique and decision making at the Halsted Memorial Training Center at Johns Hopkins Hospital.

Program director, Dr. William Roundtree's, comments: "The use of simian surrogates to perform many of the more common operations will fill a tremendous gap in the delivery of quality surgical care that was anticipated to arise over the next few years. The retirement of the huge baby boom generation threatened to put an untenable strain on the available resources. The use of chimpanzees and orangutans has, thus far, yielded outstanding results. The program is proving a point I've made for years. The many residents that have passed through these hallowed halls are no better than monkeys."

Dr. Roundtree went on to explain that originally the plan was to train baboons to provide surgical care, but it was soon discovered that all the available baboons were tied up in a sister pilot program where they were being trained to become Senators and Representatives.

The first simian surgeons are expected to complete their training in 2013, coinciding with the introduction of the first health care reforms. When asked if there was to be any role for gorillas, Dr. Roundtree remarked, "Gorillas haven't shown much aptitude for general surgery, but we are looking into training them to do orthopedics."

News of this new pilot program sent the value of Chiquita stock soaring in after hours trading today.

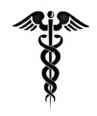

26. Surgical Education

It is predicted that over the next 10 years, as the baby boom generation ages, that there will be a shortage of available general surgeons to address the expected surgical needs of this aging population.

Recently, many general surgery residency programs have been finding it difficult to fill all their categorical positions, that is, those positions that lead to a finished general surgeon. As more and more of the population reach retirement age, it is anticipated that the incidence of GI cancers, breast cancer, peripheral vascular disease, and many other maladies prevalent among this age group will increase and there is a growing concern that the already overworked specialty of general surgery will be unable to adequately meet the challenge.

The recently passed Healthcare Reform act has squarely attacked this growing problem with several new and innovative pilot programs. The Simian Surgical project, previously reported on these pages is one such program. Another pilot program, to be headquartered in Phoenix, Arizona, is the ICS Surgical Education Program. This ground-breaking initiative, funded by an NIH grant through the recently passed healthcare bill, has as its goal to seek out highly skilled young persons and train them as surgeons. Currently, it takes many years to train a general surgeon. Four years of college, followed by four years of medical school, and then five to six years of surgery residency is the current pathway to becoming a general surgeon. The new, innovative program will streamline this pathway considerably.

Dr. Albert Scheinbach elaborates, "Recent studies suggest that highly skilled technicians can adequately perform the necessary surgery to prevent the shortfall of qualified surgeons that this country may face in the coming years. Our aim is to find the future stars of surgery at a young age, perhaps as young as nine or 10, train them in the most modern techniques, utilizing the most modern equipment available and prevent what could be tragedy for so many of our elderly."

Dr. Scheinbach explained that the initial phase will be one of recruitment. Carpet advertising in the most popular and widely read graphic journals*, as well as recruitment in various projection-oriented arcades should allow the program to find young men and women with appropriate hand-eye coordination to perform the many surgical procedures at the highest possible level. It has been clearly demonstrated that surgical skills are directly correlated to scores achieved on "Donkey Kong," Super Mario Brothers," and "Need for Speed." However, besides demonstrating the necessary hand-eye coordination, the recruitment process will also require the applicants to be able to fill out the application; the prospective surgeon will actually have to have the skill to legibly write their name and address, including postal code, on the form that will be available with the advertisement. Once accepted into the program, a vigorous, but compassionate educational and training regimen will commence.

From the comfort of their own home the student will be sent a weekly package containing the training materials, including educational manuals and anatomic parts. An instructional audio CD written by James Weldon Johnson**, famous spiritual composer, will accompany the material and will provide the student with detailed directions to allow him or her to complete the required tasks. At the end of the semester the student will be expected to return all the body parts properly assembled and fully functional. Those that pass this portion of the training will be allowed to progress to the final examination.

The final exam will be administered by the surgical staff of the University of Phoenix, International Correspondence Division, and will consist of a didactic portion as well as an actual operation. Dr. Scheinbach explains:

"The home centered education portion is not considered completely adequate training to allow our students to enter the operating theater unattended. The candidate for graduation must demonstrate the necessary dexterity to be a safe surgeon. The final exam will consist of a series of simulated procedures utilizing a standard model, Operation*** and then a computer graphics module****; successful completion of this phase is followed by an actual operation. The candidate will be assigned a random operation ranging from a simple appendectomy to a pancreatoduodenectomy. These highly skilled young people will be required to perform the assigned procedure assisted by standard operating room personnel. A grade of 70 % on this portion of the exam will be necessary to pass and be issued a diploma. The graduate will be bestowed with the degree 'Doctor of Surgery.' "

A spokesman for the Obama administration stated that the supposed complexities of most operations are exaggerated and overstated. We believe that any properly trained person, with the necessary manual dexterity and assisted by the computer modules that our team has developed, can successfully perform most of the surgery necessary for the aging baby boomer population. He added that, initially, these newly trained surgeons will provide service limited to Medi-care patients. It is anticipated that as the program becomes established and the significant cost savings are realized private insurers will jump on the bandwagon.

The initial pilot program will have 500 participants with initial training expected to be completed by January 2012.

* "Teen Titans," "Astonishing X-Men," "The Incredible Hulk," "Spiderman."

** "Dem Bones." Lyrics and music by James Weldon Johnson.

** "Operation." Hasbro toys recommended for ages 6 & up.

**** "Virtual Surgery."

Obesity is a growing health problem in the United States, an offshoot of our affluent society. Even though a portly countenance was considered a positive attribute many years ago, it is now a major health issue. Surgical intervention to treat this problem is becoming increasingly prevalent. The next two articles present alternatives to radical surgery.

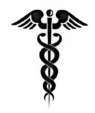

27. The Obesity Problem

The second day of a diet is always easier than the first.
By the second day you're off it.

—Jackie Gleason

Today I read an article that tried to shed light on a medical condition endemic to modern society. Obesity plagues our post modern world, particularly in the United States, and more particularly in Houston, Texas, my hometown. Houston carries the dubious distinction of having been named the least physically fit, most obese city in the US several years ago. In my general surgery practice I face this reality every day.

There is no question that obesity contributes to the rising costs of health care. Overweight patients can turn straightforward surgical conditions into complex operations that may require significant adjustment or compromise to have a successful outcome.

There is a huge industry catering to the desire of the obese individual to go from size 20 to size 8 or 48 waist to 36. Fad diets, diet pills, lap bands, and gastric bypass surgery ads fill our airways, magazines and internet pages promising a svelte and youthful body in 30 (or 60 or 90) days or your money back.

Today in surgery, while creating a colostomy (always a mind-stimulating endeavor), we proposed a powerful solution to this pervasive problem. As background let me say that human beings originally were foragers, searching for their food. Later they became hunters and eventually farmers. The scarcity of food was the driving force in ancient society and wealth was measured in sheep and cattle, rather than dollars.

Of course, times have changed and scarcity of food has become a thing of the past in our developed nations. A casual stroll down the aisle of the neighborhood megasupermarket will result in a cart laden with all the necessities of life. As a matter of fact one need not even make the short drive to the grocery. With a few clicks of your trusty mouse it is possible to select and have delivered to your front door everything you need to keep your pantry and your stomach full.

So, today, those of us in surgery decided it is time to return to our ancestral roots. The supermarket should become a place to hunt and forage for food. No longer should the shopper be allowed a leisurely stroll down capacious aisles. No, it is time to work for our food. And, to battle obesity, food that is high in fat and calories should require the greatest work. Fresh fruits and vegetables could require only a short stroll through the "Produce Patch." However, high fat steaks would need to be hunted, perhaps in a way akin to laser tag, requiring shooting a moving freezer to claim the elusive porterhouse. A craving for donuts would necessitate rock climbing a 40-foot wall and Twinkies would oblige the shopper to face a fire-breathing dragon, armed only with a sword and a shield.

This very modest plan would fight obesity in several ways. The effort expended to successfully reach the desired food would burn off a considerable number of calories. Those individuals that are unable to put forth the necessary effort would have to forego their fried pork rinds or Ben and Jerry's and be forced to diet or eat healthy, easily obtainable food.

This plan could solve not only the problem of obesity, but also food shortages in some countries as extra, unobtainable food would become available and could be shipped to those in need. A major healthcare issue also would be addressed and in the long term health care costs would go down. Such a modest change could reap benefits for decades.

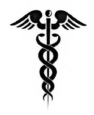

28. Voodooweightloss.com

I've been on a diet for two weeks and all I've lost is two weeks.

—Totie Fields

If you are overweight and want a quick and easy way to slim down then checkout Voodooweightloss.com. This remarkable diet plan is guaranteed to help you shed those unwanted pounds in a matter of weeks and all with a minimum of effort on your part. Too good to be true? Of course, it sounds like voodoo and, the amazing thing is, IT IS VOODOO.

That's right. Madame Marie, Queen of the Voodoo curse, straight from Haiti, the voodoo capital of the world, guarantees that if you follow her plan you will be a size two in no time. Even better, Voodooweightloss.com's weight loss program allows you to eat anything and everything. I know what you're thinking: This is some kind of scam. But, the tried and true voodoo methods, perfected over thousands of years, are now available for your dieting pleasure.

Madame Marie will use her skills to slowly slim your hips, tighten your thighs and arms, firm your chin, eliminate that unsightly cellulite, and, for a small extra fee, enhance your breasts and buttocks. For you male customers, she can give you six pack abs, rock hard biceps, a tight shapely butt, and a sharp, chiseled face. Other enhancements may also be available (extra fees may apply).

How does she do it? Is it magic? No, it's voodoo. For a brief time we are offering Madame's amazing service at the incredibly low introductory price of $69.95. For this initial low fee a miniature voodoo doll will be constructed in proper proportion to your current body habitus. Madame Marie, employing secret Voodoo techniques known to only a few Voodoo High Priestesses, will, over a period of several weeks, gradually mold your likeness into a svelte image of the self you want to be. Want to be Barbie? She can do it. Rush jobs are available for an extra fee.

So, if you have a class reunion coming up and want to show that bully from high school what you're really made of, give Madame a buzz. She will turn those thunder thighs into tight, muscular limbs that will make you the envy of every man and woman that ever made fun of you.

Just send $69.95, plus $12.95 to cover the cost of the dead chicken, along with any personal item (Fine jewelry preferred) to www.voodoooweightloss.com and start to see the pounds melt away.

Disclaimer: Not approved by the American Academy of Weight Loss Programs. Once the contract is signed all obligations must be fulfilled. The Voodoo Weight Loss program can also work in reverse. Individual results may vary.

American Express, Mastercard, Visa, and Paypal accepted.

Obesity is a problem that pervades our society. In medicine and, particularly surgery, whenever there are a large number of techniques for a particular operation it is generally accepted that none of them is perfect and each has a drawback or flaw. The number of diet programs available suggests that there is no one program that works better than any other. The glycemic advantage, low carb high fiber, high carb low fat, high fat low carb, Atkins, South Beach, Jenny, and all the others all seem like voodoo to me. Proper diet and exercise, although archaic and requiring some determination by the individual, are the keys to safe and effective weight loss. But if you are looking for a safe, albeit unorthodox weight loss program, check out Madame Marie and Voodooweightloss.com.

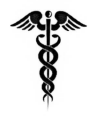

29. *Fashion Statements*

Fashion is all about happiness. It's fun. It's important. But it's not medicine.

—Donatella Versace

I reside in the world of surgery where fashion is rarely much of a consideration. The isolation of the operating theater does not lend itself to making fashion statements. When I first entered private practice 20 years ago, I always started my day wearing a dress shirt and tie underneath my white lab coat. Most of the time the professional look was quickly replaced by surgical scrub suits and I found myself changing back and forth three or four times a day. So, the shirt and tie faded away, permanently replaced by scrub suits.

Initially, I wore whatever scrub suit I pulled from my closet where a varied arsenal of scrubs "borrowed" from almost every hospital I'd ever frequented was housed. These scrubs ranged from blue to gray to various shades of green. The scrubs from Strong Memorial Hospital in Rochester, New York had a peculiar feature in that the material was 55% cotton, 44% polyester, and 1% stainless steel. I always assumed that the 1% was woven throughout the fabric, but it would have been more prudent to concentrate it in certain strategic areas, given the demeanor of some of the surgical attending staff at that hospital.

The cheapest scrubs were those from Nassau County Medical Center, where I did a portion of my surgical residency. White scrubs with pink "NCMC" stamped all over and pretty much see-through guaranteed that no one would ever wear a pair out in public. Actually, many did not even want to wear them in the OR, unless one wished to advertise certain assets. These have sat on my shelf for years, but were useful when I was painting our living room with the help of my kids. For some unknown reason I had several scrubs in size small which were perfect covering for my young helpers.

Surgical scrubs, until recently, were never designed to be anything but functional. Loose and drab, they could never be considered flattering. But, to rescue us from the drab and dreary, come designer scrubs. It seems there was an anesthesiology resident that tackled this problem head on and created her own line of designer (overpriced) scrub suits. As has been done with blue jeans, she added some stitching on the pockets, made them a bit more form fitting and, thus, more flattering; creating a product that has allowed her to give up medicine and become a fashion mogul. Smart move with "healthcare reform" looming large on the horizon.

The other item of surgical clothing that lends itself to fashion statements is the surgical cap. These come in quite a variety of styles. Nurses typically wear the bouffant type, billowy and comfortable. Other types are the tie around skull cap and surgical hoods. Most male surgeons favor the tied skull cap, while personnel that sport beards usually opt for the improved coverage of the hood. Many of our nursing personnel make their own head covering, adding a touch of color or whimsy to the usual drab décor. Personally, I am in the minority of surgeons it seems, because I prefer to wear the bouffant style of head covering. Besides the superior coverage which, theoretically, will decrease the risk of contaminating the operative field, these hats are more comfortable. Never sacrifice comfort for style, I always say, much to my wife's consternation.

Of course, there is more to surgical fashion than scrub suits and caps. Consider our patients. Certain bodily adornments are unique to the surgical patient. In particular, wound dressings, drains, scars, and the ubiquitous exam gown adorn the surgical patient.

Modern surgery has evolved to its present state of ambulatory procedures, short hospital stays, and rapid return to normal activity. This is all for the best and, ultimately, improves patient outcome. But, a consequence to these advances is the necessity to send patients home with freshly dressed incisions, surgical drains, and sometimes open wounds that require daily care.

In the old days, circa 1980, surgical patients remained in the hospital until they had enough time to enjoy significant healing. Specifically, it was routine to keep the patient in the hospital until any and all drains were removed. This could mean overnight or two weeks. Indeed, it was a frequent response at surgical conferences, when asked why a patient was still in the hospital, to answer that they still had a drain.

Times have changed, however, and patients routinely are discharged after their outpatient laparoscopic cholecystectomy or removal of soft tissue mass or breast tumor with some sort of drain. These are almost always of the class called "closed suction" drains, a fenestrated or perforated plastic end that sits within the operative site connected to another plastic tube that is tunneled under the skin and exits through an opening in the skin at a location some distance from the wound. The tunneled tube is connected to some sort of self suction apparatus; commonly a hollow bulb that is squeezed flat and provides a source of suction as it recoils to its normal state. Such a drain removes fluids that would otherwise accumulate in the surgical and wound and helps promote proper healing.

However, the patient is left with a dilemma, of sorts. How does one carry such a device in a way that is inconspicuous, functional, and comfortable. At least the designers gave a bit of thought to this problem. The collection bulbs (what I call the "hand grenade" because of its shape) has a tab around its neck that allows it to be safety pinned to an article of clothing. So, most commonly the drainage system is pinned to a shirt or some other article of clothing or put in a pocket, often discreetly visible but not particularly noticeable.

Some patients are far more inventive. A favorite of female patients, particularly those that are amply endowed, is to stuff the drainage bulb into their bra. This keeps it well hidden, but also makes for some adventurous searching on rounds or in the office when it is necessary to check the effluent for quantity and quality. Similarly, male patients will occasionally carry it in their underwear; this works best with briefs rather than boxers.

Wound dressings generally require little attention and are rarely subject to invention. Most often they are white gauze and tape, left in place for 48 hours and simply removed. However, open wounds may require that the patient wear the dressing for weeks and sometimes months. Surgical gauze can be expensive and many patients opt for low cost alternatives. The most common is a feminine hygiene pad of some sort, sterile, absorbent, and well-suited to the task. Understandably, these are usually utilized for wounds that are out of the public eye.

Alternatives include cloth towels of variable cleanliness, paper towels, adhesive tape by itself, and frequently nothing.

It is remarkable that so many wounds heal perfectly well in spite of the lack of attention they receive; a testament to the wonderful healing capabilities that are built into our bodies.

Finally, there are exam gowns; a garment that is designed for only one purpose: to make the wearer look and feel as foolish as possible. Hospital gowns are designed with a variety of ties and snaps purportedly to make it easier to examine the patient. But, it is common for these gowns to cause the most learned academician's blood pressure to rise as he struggles to undo the numerous ties which are invariably knotted and usually lead even the most rational doctor to rip or cut the offensive garment, and then exclaim, "I guess the hospital can send me a bill." For the patient the gowns leave them open and exposed and many will sport two to provide complete coverage and not to reveal their "assets" to an entire ward.

In my office we have paper gowns, cheap, somewhat cumbersome, but adequate. These gowns do have one unique feature. They come with a plastic "belt." I think that this belt was designed by a runway model as it is only about twenty four inches long. Usually I find it on the floor of the exam room, sometimes the patient will be holding it with a very confused look on his or her face. Once in a while someone will actually try to put it on and one creative man tied it around his head, similar to a famous painting, a trophy to the scars he had suffered in the course of his surgery.

Therefore, the next time you watch celebrities queuing up on the red carpet being interviewed and asked, "Who are you wearing," think about the fashion statements made by the medical profession, perhaps not very glamorous, but certainly creative.

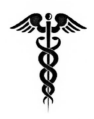

30. *It's Alimentary*

Character is higher than intellect.
——Ralph Waldo Emerson

My recent work has taken me to weaving my way in and around people's bowels, something that is a common task for any general surgeon. However, I've had more than my usual share over the last few weeks. While making my way around a particularly difficult colon today, those of us in the operating room discussed the relative merits of what has been named the alimentary tract, our intestines, the gastrointestinal tract, bowel, guts, or "chitlins."

If one considers all of our various organs one would have to agree that our GI tract is, by far, the most intelligent. Think about it, our brain stands isolated within its protective cage, so snobby and aloof, only allowing certain special materials to enter its domain, always giving orders, but out of touch with its co-organs. The heart is a tireless worker, but mindlessly does the same thing over and over, day in and day out, blood comes in, blood goes out. Ditto for the lungs, a monotonous pastime of breath in, breath out, inhale, exhale, occasionally fending off noxious fumes and fighting invaders.

Kidneys are efficient cleaners and bones are glorified coat racks. Muscle is a little smarter, only working when called upon, but always the same thing, relax, then contract, hold this up, push that down. No wonder they get stiff and sore.

But our bowels do remarkable things. When not needed they rest, blood flow is shut down, and our guts essentially go to sleep. Yet, when called upon, they spring into action, sorting out a variety of nutrients, directing them to the liver through the bloodstream or bypassing the liver, sending fats through our lymphatic system.

This long tunnel through the middle of our body is constantly fending off invaders, be they micro-organisms, noxious chemicals, or a variety of foreign bodies. The GI tract lives in symbiosis with huge numbers of bacteria, using these microscopic invaders for its (and our) own purpose. Yet, if one of these foreigners behaves badly they are expelled, one way or another, causing us a brief period of discomfort, but also keeping us well. No other organ has to deal with such insults on so massive a scale, yet our bowels handle them with aplomb. Perhaps, our skin, the body's largest organ, comes close, but on a much smaller scale.

And, our bowels can learn. Remove the stomach and replace it with a segment of small intestine and this small intestine will learn to be the stomach, stretching to accommodate our food, adapting to its new role like an understudy filling in for the stricken star.

So, I say, let us praise our bowels. When they are working properly they keep us happy, healthy, and whole. But, when they go bad; when they are blocked or punctured or dying, nothing can make us so incredibly ill. I say there should be a take your bowel to lunch day. But, come to think of it, everyday is take your bowel to lunch day.

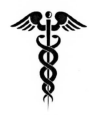

31. Why . . . a Surgeon?

What do I do for a living? I save lives and stamp out disease.

—David Gelber, MD

I f you've made it this far I hope the question above has been answered for you. At the end of medical school a decision is made; the decision to choose what type of doctor the student wants to become. I debated between pediatrics and surgery, opposite ends of the spectrum, and in the end I decided that surgery was a better fit for me.

I've spent years attending to the drunks who couldn't settle their differences without knives or guns, children with an appendix that decided to burst at 2:00 a.m., kindly old ladies who've said, "I'm done with those old breasts, just get rid of them," and on and on. The rewards are tremendous, but at what price? The patients come first and, although I've tried the best I can, family life has suffered. Is it worth it? Nearly every week I can look back and say that I saved somebody's life, stopped their bleeding, removed their cancer, restored their ability to walk without pain or disability,

Nights of no sleep, hours standing at an operating room table, sitting at a bedside until I'm satisfied that everything is OK, sitting and explaining over and over until the patient understands, is comfortable and confident that they are going to receive the best care I can give, have given me a great personal satisfaction. Over the years I've taken care of some of the finest people I've ever met and some who are not so fine. But, no matter, I've tried to give all of them my utmost skill, attention and care.

Why a surgeon? I hope you've learned the answer after reading these words.

Glossary of Common Terms

Aerodigestive Tract: the upper digestive tract and airways, including mouth, pharynx (throat), trachea, and bronchi (windpipes).

Anastamosis: surgically connected one organ to another, usually involving portions of the gastrointestinal tract or blood vessels.

Anesthesia: the process of numbing and relaxing the body or a part of the body which allows surgery to be performed. Anesthesia is usually administered by an Anesthesiologist (physician) or an Anesthetist (nurse or assistant).

Angiogenesis: the ingrowth of new blood vessels which is an important component of the healing process. Angiogenesis also can be associated with the growth of tumors.

Aortic aneurysm: a weakened area on the aorta, the largest artery in the body which can burst and cause sudden death; rupture of an aortic aneurysm is always a life-threatening surgical emergency.

Appendectomy: surgery to remove the appendix.

Appendicitis: inflammation of the appendix, a common condition that requires surgery.

Appendix: a wormlike structure that arises from the cecum, the first part of the large intestine; it frequently becomes inflamed causing appendicitis.

Asepsis: sterile technique, important for preventing infections during surgery.

Cholecystectomy: surgery to remove the gallbladder.

Cholecystitis: inflammation of the gallbladder.

Cholelithiasis: gallstones, usually composed of cholesterol or bilirubin, components of bile which is stored in the gallbladder.

Coagulopathy: a condition where blood does not clot normally.

Dialysis: artificially cleaning the blood for patients with kidney failure.

Diverticulitis: inflammation of diverticuli, small outpouchings from the intestine, usually from the large intestine (colon).

Diverticulosis: outpouchings from the intestine, most common in the large intestine.

Electrocautery: device that utilizes electrical energy to seal blood vessels.

Enteral: given into the gastrointestinal tract.

Gangrene: death of tissue or an organ caused by lack of adequate blood supply.

Fistula: an abnormal connection between two organs, usually involving drainage of secretions from one of the organs into the other. Fistulas may be the result of poor healing after surgery.

Hematoma: a localized collection of clotted blood.

Hemorrhoids: veins around the anus that act as cushions; they can bleed, enlarge, and protrude, or thrombose and cause severe pain.

Hemorrhoidectomy: surgery to remove hemorrhoids.

Hernia: a weak area in the abdominal wall that allows protrusion of intraabdominal organs; a very common condition that can cause discomfort, disability, and can only be repaired with surgery.

Hiatal Hernia: the passage of intraabdominal organs through the esophageal hiatus into the chest, commonly causing gastric reflux. Usually repaired laparoscopically.

Intensive Care Unit (ICU): a nursing unit in a hospital that provides specialized care to very ill patients.

Imaging: techniques available to see inside the body, such as x-rays, CT scans, MRI, ultrasound, and PET scan.

Laparoscopy: surgical technique utilizing tiny incisions and a high resolution camera and monitor.

Microorganism: bacteria, virus, parasite, or fungus that can infect the body. Bacteria are of greatest concern in surgery.

Minimally Invasive: surgical technique that allows an operation to be done with tiny or no incision, such as laparoscopy or arthroscopy.

Necrosis: infection within dead tissue, often foul smelling and draining pus.

Omentum: an apron of fat and blood vessels that lies superficial to our abdominal organs.

Pancreatitis: inflammation of the pancreas.

Parenteral: given to the whole body, usually through a vein.

Pressor: medicine given to help maintain acceptable blood pressure, may be inotropic, which increases the strength of heart contractions or chronotropic, which increases heartrate.

Sepsis: a severe, systemic infection that is life threatening, frequently caused by conditions that require emergency surgery, such as gangrene of an organ.

Suture: threadlike material that is used in surgery to sew things together. Some suture is designed to dissolve after a few days, weeks, or months, while others are permanent.

Vascular Surgery: surgery on blood vessels.

Ventilator/Respirator: a machine that assumes the task of breathing for patients who are too ill to breathe on their own or unable to breathe because they are undergoing surgery or have suffered severe trauma/illness.

Acknowledgements

I wish to thank Gianna Carini and Duncan Long for their help in publishing *Behind the Mask.*

About the Author

Dr. David Gelber has been in private practice in General Surgery for more than 20 years in the Houston, Texas, area. He is a partner in Coastal Surgical Group and prior to this he was Chief of the Trauma Service and Director of the Surgical Intensive Care Unit at Nassau County Medical Center on Long Island in New York.

He is Board Certified in General Surgery and Surgical Critical Care and is a Fellow of the American College of Surgeons. He was named one of "America's Top Doc's" by Castle Connolly for 2008. His other published works are "Future Hope, ITP Book One" and "Joshua and Aaron, ITP Book Two"; religious science fiction novels. More of his writing can be found on his blog, "Heard in the OR" at heardintheor.blogspot.com.

He has been married to Laura for twenty five years and has three children, four dogs, and numerous birds.